SIMPLY
GLUTEN-FREE

SIMPLY
GLUTEN-FREE

Rita Greer's helpful kitchen handbook

Rita Greer

SOUVENIR PRESS

Contents

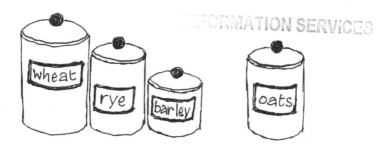

CHAPTER 1

Gluten-Free –
What Does it Mean?

What is gluten?
Gluten is a transparent, rubbery, sticky protein found in wheat, rye and barley. A different kind is found in oats, called avenin – more about that later. Gluten is what enables us to bake shaped bread, make cakes that will hold up fruit, crisp biscuits, pastry, thickened soups and sauces and baking that doesn't just fall into a heap of crumbs. **Gluten holds things together and smooths things out.** It has been in man's diet for thousands of years. The best gluten is in wheat and most of us eat it several times a day without even noticing it. We are nourished by it, but, for some it is banned from the diet and for them a gluten-free diet is essential.

What does 'a gluten free diet' mean?
Quite simply, it means a different lifestyle of eating food without any gluten containing grains. There are no pills to

help so it has to be a particular diet without wheat, rye, barley (and possibly oats) as all these contain gluten. If people who shouldn't be eating gluten continue to eat it on a regular basis they can become very ill and stay ill, or worse.

Up to the middle of the 20th century, nothing was understood about gluten making chidren and adults unwell and could even cause them to die prematurely because they kept on eating gluten, unaware it was the cause of their deteriorating health. Babies who had been healthy on a diet of milk did not thrive when weaned and given solid food which contained gluten. It was all very tragic, inexplicable and mysterious. You can see, for some people a gluten-free diet is not just a silly fad. These people need it for their very survival.

When it was first discovered, after the second world war, that some people who had been denied wheat did much better without it and then became worse again when it came back into their diet. White coated men in laboratories answer to the problem was to take the gluten out of wheat and just use the starch for 'bread'. This particular bread was mainly distributed through pharmacies and prescribed by a medical practitioners in UK. It was kept out of sight of the general public and it wasn't allowed to be advertised or displayed. It wasn't until years later that women in aprons in domestic kitchens got to work on the practical side of the problem that things began to change. Blends with a mixture of naturally gluten-free starches and a binder were designed to mimic wheat. There was a great effort to make the lot of the gluten-free dieter better and cookery books began to appear. By the 21st century this kind of exclusion diet necessary for coeliacs (pronounced see-lee-acks) was being used by others suffering a variety of complaints – MS, IBS, arthritis, dermatitis, ME, allergies, bloating, some kinds of arthritis etc. Because the special gluten-free food is eaten at home the medical profession has no real control over it, so it is not like taking prescribed pills. More people adopt a gluten-free diet by their own choice than people medically diagnosed and advised to do it. Providing a sensible, balanced gluten-free diet is enjoyed, such a diet is no threat to anyone's health. Millions of people, all over the globe are on such a diet quite by accident because they live in countries where wheat is not the main source of food.

Invisible problem
Who would have thought there was any harm in eating bread for some people? Unfortunately, there is and it is not just bread but everything made with wheat flour –- rolls, scones, pastry, cakes, biscuits, pasta etc. – the obvious food made with wheat flour. And it isn't just wheat, it is barley and rye too and maybe oats. The main problem with wheat flour (which contains gluten) is, because it has such useful and amazing properties, it finds its way into a lot of manufactured foods for various reasons such as thickening sauces and coating food before frying, making mixtures smooth and combining with other weaker flours. Ordinary wheat flour is made stronger to give better baking results by adding extra gluten. There seems to be no escape.

(A word here about rice as it is described as 'glutinous'. Note the spelling 'in' instead of 'en'. Glutinous merely means sticky. It doesn't mean there is gluten in rice.)

Gluten pops up where least expected and you can't see it or taste it. Its presence is not obvious and it doesn't have to be used in large quantities to cause trouble to a gluten-free dieter. The food industry loves it. It needs keeping an eye on, especially when manufacturers suddenly change their formulas. Think of it as an *invisible enemy*.

Contamination
There is also the problem of contamination. Sometimes foods which are actually gluten-free are processed and packed in

factories where gluten- containing foods are also processed and packed, allowing gluten to get into them.

Naturally gluten-free food

Fortunately, there are many kinds of food which are naturally gluten-free. It is no coincidence that most of them are unprocessed. In a healthy diet they will make up over three quarters of what you eat. Here they are.

All fresh and frozen *plain fruit*
All fresh and frozen *plain vegetables*
All fresh and frozen *plain meat, poultry*
All fresh and frozen *plain fish and shellfish*
All fresh *eggs*
All plain *cheeses*
All fresh *milk, butter and cream*
Most *margarines*; sunflower, maize, extra virgin olive, soya, safflower *oils*
(Avoid margarines and salad dressings with wheatgerm oil.)

The problem foods are that other one quarter – bread, cakes, biscuits, pasta, crispbreads, scones, cookies, pastries, crumpets, buns, pancakes, pastry, crumble toppings, breakfast cereals, confectionery, cake decorations, chutney, table sauces, some canned vegetables, bedtime drinks, soups – the list goes on … Food in packets, in cans, on the shelves, in the freezers. These are the foods that need to be replaced with gluten-free versions and these are the foods that demand a different lifestyle. You can see by the basic list they are mostly foods with a high level of carbohydrate. A new gluten-free diet will mean gluten-free carbohydrates. Don't panic! Rice, potatoes, sweetcorn and bananas are all high in carbohydrates and are widely available. In their natural form they are all gluten-free. There are others in the form of flours – rice flour, cornflour, potato flour and gram (chickpea) flour. All these are naturally gluten-free too. There are others which are not so easy to come by. However, none of them can be said to be completely gluten-free if they have been contaminated by wheat/rye/barley and possibly oats during processing/storage or packaging.

Thickeners etc
Although the situation has improved regarding labeling of ingredients, manufacturers on the whole are not geared to the gluten-free dieter –- there are not enough of them to worry about. Any of the following listed on a product *might* mean gluten as they don't make it clear. **If in doubt avoid.**

flour, thickener, rusk
special edible starch, modified starch, food starch
corn, starch, *cornflour/cornstarch, cereal
binding, binder, cereal protein, edible starch,
vegetable protein, MSG, wheat glucose-sucrose.
MSG is a flavour enhancer which can be made from several things, including wheat.
**‘Corn’ in some countries means any kind of grain, not just maize. When buying cornflour always check that it is maize and not some other grain.*

Here is a list of ingredients that are made from wheat/rye/ barley or oats. (This book is not just for coeliacs but for people who need to avoid all contact with wheat, rye and barley and oats. The jury is still out on oats for some people. See chapter 14 for more information on oats.)

Ingredients/foods made from grains that contain gluten

wheat bran, wheat flour, wheat berries, wheatmeal, wheat protein, wheat starch

wholewheat, cracked wheat, kibbled wheat, durum wheat,
    wheat fructose-sucrose, wheatgerm, wheatgerm oil
semolina
couscous
pourgouri
burghul, bulghar, bulgar wheat
granary flour
rye meal, rye flour, rye flakes
barley meal, barley flour, pearl barley, barley flakes,
    pot barley, barley malt
malt vinegar, malt

Oats *(contain avenin, a kind of protein similar, but not the
same as gluten).*
oats, porridge oats, rolled oats, jumbo oats, oat flakes, oat-
bran, oatgerm, oatmeal, pinhead oatmeal, medium and fine
oatmeal, oatmilk

Caution
Gluten **might** be in the following. Annoyingly, it might not.
You need to check labels before you buy and use. Always
check to avoid a mistake.

baby foods, baked beans, baking powder, batter and
pancake mixes, biscuits and biscuit mixes, blancmange,
breakfast cereals, burgers
cakes, cake mixes, chocolate, chocolates, chutney, cocoa,
drinking chocolate, coffee (cheap brands), communion
wafers, corned beef, cornflour (cornstarch),cream (non-
dairy), crispbreads, crisps (flavoured)
crumble topping mix, curry powder, custard (ready-made),
custard powder
mayonnaise, meat with stuffing/coatings, muesli, made
mustard

pancakes, pancake mixes, pastas, pastry, pastry mixes,
pepper (white, catering)
pickles, pie fillings, porridge, potato (instant), puddings
salad dressings, sandwich spreads, sauces, sausages, snack
nibbles, soups (mixes/tins/packets) soy sauce, spaghetti,
spreads, desserts/instant puddings, fish in crumbs/
batter/coatings, gravy powder/mixes, ice cream, macaroni,
malt, sprouted grains, stock cubes/powder/ pastes, pâtés,
stuffing, mixes for stuffing,
suet, sweets, flavoured yoghurts

*Because gluten can appear in all these you need to read the
labels and to find gluten-free versions if there are any, otherwise make them yourself at home. Sometimes there are not
any labels to read and this requires knowledge and caution.*
Freshly ground black pepper is safest. (A catering estab-
lishment trick is to stretch white pepper with wheat flour.) You
can buy small, pocket-sized grinders for black pepper to carry
around with you from good kitchen shops.)
  *Some coeliacs and allergics also have a problem with lac-
tose which is found in milk. There are several kinds of
lactose-free milks and products on the market. You will find
these at the supermarket or health store.*

Reading the ingredients boxes on products
Some packets and tins are so small the print needs to be read
with a magnifying glass. Buy a pocket size one from an opti-
cians. (This isn't a joke, I mean it.) There are all kinds of rules
and regulations about labeling and gluten-free comes under
this legislation. If a food has more than 20 parts per million
of gluten it cannot be labeled as 'gluten free'. Between 21
parts and 100 parts per million, foods have to be labelled
'very low gluten'. Something called the Codex Alimentarius
allows *wheat starch* for a gluten-free diet for coeliacs. This

would not be good for a wheat allergic and it is hardly nourishing or easy to use. After processing out as much of the gluten as possible it is still not completely gluten free. In spite of this it is legal to label it 'gluten-free'. For foods that might be contaminated with gluten there are strict codes. These are not deliberately contaminated in some hate campaign, it just happens during processing and packing when they are done on the same premises. Manufacturers cannot be expected to maintain special dedicated premises and machinery just for the gluten-free community, which forms only a small part of the total population. Manufacturers are in a difficult position, especially those who export to the UK. Some of them are frightened of being sued and prefer to just put 'not suitable for a gluten-free diet'. or 'may contain ...' This is an easy option for them. Increased regulation seems to be leading to manufacturers being put off being helpful and they mainly have to be trusted to tell the truth on their packaging, as there is no army of inspectors going around testing their products. Gluten-free dieters will only ever be a small percentage of the population and this has to be faced.

Most people have no understanding of the practical problems of a gluten-free diet. A good example of this is the problem of communion wafers. At one time there was no such thing as gluten-free communion wafers. Now there are, often a different shape such as square. When these are offered at communion they can often be mixed together on the communion plate.

Contamination control
In bakeries, food production units and mills where wheat is processed there is a great deal of flour with gluten. It hangs into the air in a sort of mist, it gets all over everything – staff overalls, under their fingernails and on their skin. To avoid

contamination there would have to be a 'dedicated' unit away from the source of contamination with different staff and a completely different environment. The costs would be enormous. It is recognized as a problem to allergics as manufacturers are now inclined to put cautions on their products, warning allergics not to eat them rather than take the risk. Sesame seeds, nuts and wheat seem to be the main offenders which can be processed, packed and stored in an undedicated factory. Gluten-free dieters would be wise to heed this kind of warning.

At home, in the kitchen, the risk of contamination is high if food is not kept separate, with dedicated aprons, baking tins, a dedicated toaster reserved exclusively for gluten-free toast and baking and handling food with clean hands and fingernails. Wheat flour dust is a problem. If you start baking in a clean kitchen and you have both gluten-free and wheat baking to do, tackle the gluten-free first before wheat contamination can take place. As soon as food is cold it can be wrapped in food film. Dedicated containers for biscuits, cakes and bread are necessary and storage space in the kitchen for gluten-free food should be separate from the rest of the kitchen.

See chapter 14 for different approaches to coping with a gluten-free diet as there are more ways than one of dealing with it. Choose one to suit your way of life.

Take some comfort from the list of naturally gluten-free foods. If you feel you ought to lean in that direction you could be on the verge of going over to a much healthier diet either for yourself or the person for whom you are providing food.

A healthy gluten-free diet could be the best news you could ever have as it will stop you eating thousands of junkfoods!

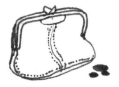

CHAPTER 2

Shopping, Kitchen Cupboard and Equipment

Shopping

With a gluten-free diet in the house, shopping will not be the same. If you are trying to buy a somewhat obscure product, telephone or E-mail supermarkets or health food stores. Go on the internet to find alternative suppliers if you can. You may have to buy in more than you need right away so as not to run out if a regular supply is not possible.

If a product says 'store in a cool dry place' it doesn't mean the fridge.

Some items you will be able to buy on your usual shopping expedition– fresh or frozen meat and fish, vegetables and fruit. If you are shopping in a large supermarket there will probably be a 'free from' section with quite a number of items marked 'gluten-free'. (Some will definitely not be gluten-free.) Study the prices. They will be higher in price than ordinary food so choose carefully and avoid buying too much.

Supermarkets are more interested in you buying finished products, not the raw materials for baking your own gluten-free items at home. They know homemade is cheaper.

If you think for a moment there could be confusion in your own kitchen about what is gluten-free and what isn't, it is a good idea to mark products and ingredients with a sticker, especially when the new regime begins. An office shop will have tiny stickers, otherwise use stick-on address labels and write on them by hand, including the date. For the freezer you will need a special pen that can cope with writing being frozen and one which will write on plastic bags.

Here is a list of the new ingredients you may need. ('Large' packs for gluten-free cooking are quite small in comparison with wheat flour.)

Starches to replace wheat

Potato flour – sometimes called 'farina' – supermarket 'free from' section or health store – buy 2 large packs.

Gram flour – this is made from chickpeas – supermarket 'free from' section or health store – buy a large pack.

Cornflour (pure maize) (large carton)– supermarket baking section or health store – buy 2 large packs.

Rice flour – health store or supermarket 'free-from' section – buy 2 large packs

Ground rice – a coarse kind of rice flour. Make sure you buy one from a dedicated mill/factory. One pack will last you ages.

(Other starches such as millet flour, tapioca flour, sago, arrowroot and buckwheat are gluten-free but I have not used them in this handbook.) Buckwheat is interesting because it is not really a wheat as it belongs to the rhubarb family. It is usually milled and packed in the same mills as wheat. (Its other name is Saracen corn.)

Binders to replace gluten

Xanthan gum – health store or supermarket 'free from' section – buy 1 drum – it lasts ages. See note on page 23.
jam-sugar-with-pectin – supermarket sugar section – buy 1 pack. This can only be used when a recipe requires sugar but it is useful for cakes and has a very clean taste.
egg white – readily available and inexpensive
apple – fresh or stewed will contain pectin
(There are other binders such as guar gum and methylcellulose but I have not used them in this handbook.)

Gluten-free breakfast cereals

If you want to use gluten-free breakfast cereals these will be flagged as gluten-free. Some supermarkets have their own brand. A health store or a 'free from' section in a large super-market will have a selection – at a price. Just buy one to start with to see if they are acceptable. Avoid buying several different ones at once as you will have to find somewhere to put them and they take up a lot of space. The ones to look for are mostly based on corn and rice, not wheat.

Fresh and frozen food

Your fresh and frozen fruit and vegetables and fresh and frozen meat and fish – all gluten-free – can be bought when you do the family shop.

Stock

If you want to use a stock cube for stock, find a suitable one that is gluten-free – it will say so on the carton – and a gluten-free Tamari-type soy sauce. Products with a short list of ingredients are better than ones with a long list. These will be in the cooking sections of the supermarket. (You will need a magnifying glass.) Your health store will probably be able to get in the special soy sauce if they don't already stock it. (Beware unscrupulous brands just called Tamari as a selling point.) The real tamari type soy sauce is thickened with rice. The others are thickened with wheat and are not gluten-free. Check labels carefully. It keeps for years so don't be afraid to buy more than one. It is very useful as stock as it has so few ingredients, unlike stock cubes which can have a whole legion of ingredients. Health stores and 'free from' sections in supermarkets are the best place to find one to suit you.

Cooking and baking trends
By the end of the last century, the media had become obsessed with celebrity chefs and cooks, coffee table cookbooks were the norm and the plot had been well and truly lost regarding food. It had drifted away from the idea of eating to sustain life and keep healthy. Feasting and entertainment became the core of food. Kitchens followed this. Batteries of expensive gadgets that take ages to wash up and gadgets that will perform what a sharp knife or two will accomplish easily with skill. Homecooks have been overwhelmed by this attitude and have become deskilled and lacking in confidence. Kitchen shops and stores have shelves of silly tools and people buy them to ape the celebrity chefs and cooks. This is not what cooking is about. You do not need lots of kitchen gadgets, merely a few useful tools. What you do need is to build your skill and confidence. There is nothing difficult about gluten-free cooking. Anyone can do it if they work at it. There is no need to spend a fortune in the kitchen shops. Here is a basic list for a gluten-free kitchen.

Kitchen tools and equipment
You will need a patty tin and cake papers for making buns.
    If you want to make muffins you will need a muffin tin with muffin papers. Supermarkets will have these, or kitchen shops.

A small loaf tin ½ lb (¼ kilo) might be difficult to buy, as will an old fashioned 1lb (500g) loaf tin, but a good kitchen shop will probably be able to help, or try the Internet. Cake tins and sponge tins are needed with baking trays and a baking sheet. You probably have a rolling pin and a wire cooling rack but separate ones for gluten-free cooking might be a good idea. Buy a roll of baking parchment, a roll of greaseproof paper and a large roll of food film for wrapping. A mini food processor is useful for making breadcrumbs and pâtés and for grinding nuts.

A blender is useful for liquidizing soups and making mayonnaise.

A stainless steel mouli is a hand tool and will make soups in a gentler way so that you can get a coarse, medium or smooth texture. (It is also much quieter than the ear-splitting electronic blitz of the blender.)

A wire mesh strainer and a colander, a steamer with a lid that will fit over a saucepan is needed for vegetables.

A stainless steel hand grater, which is sharp and easy to hold while you grate, is essential.

Bowls and basins, wooden spoons, biscuit cutters, metal skewers, saucepans, a heavy based frying pan, a griddle if you can afford one, omelet pan and a coated pan for making sauces, a cutting board that is easy to wash up, a large knife, a good breadknife with a serrated edge and a really good, small kitchen knife and kitchen scissors, a simple wooden rolling pin, scales, 2 clockwork timers (invaluable – buy from supermarkets) a set of measuring spoons and a clearly marked measuring jug are probably all you want, apart from an oven.

There is no need for your kitchen to look like a laboratory with expensive gadgets. Except for the mini-processor, blender and clockwork timers, just simple hand tools that feel comfortable and enable you to develop skills are all that are required.

You will need some kitchen tools only for use in making

gluten-free food particularly wooden spoons and a pastry brush. You can mark these on the end of the handles with a blob of coloured nail varnish. They should be kept just for gluten-free cooking and not ever used for wheat cooking.

Ovens
There are all kinds of ovens, all different sizes, for gas, electricity and with fans etc. I can only give you a clue as to what shelf height is required and what Gas setting and temperatures Centigrade and Farenheit to use. Fan ovens will need working out from the instruction book. The recipes are just a guide and the ones I use for my own perfectly ordinary oven in a domestic kitchen. You will probably need to adjust slightly one way or the other. Make notes in the margin if your oven differs. (You know your own oven but I don't have that advantage.) Microwaves are not ovens for cooking but merely warming food up and defrosting quickly. They are not meant for baking. Second hand shops, car boot and garage sales, and charity shops can be a good source of second hand kitchen equipment. Kitchen shops and department stores are a good source of new equipment and a lot of silly gadgets.

Safety in the kitchen
Kitchens can be dangerous places with blood, fire, boiling water, sharp knives, hot ovens and flaming hobs as well as a wet floor to slip on. Try to do everything at a measured pace instead of rushing. It is easy to get burnt and to cut yourself.

When using knives, concentrate on what you are doing. Don't allow yourself to get distracted. Wear oven gloves for taking things out of the oven. If you spill something on the floor, wipe it up immediately. Don't leave tea towels near flames so that they catch fire. Don't put oil into a pan and heat it unattended. A packet of plasters and a tube of burn ointment in the kitchen drawer will come in handy.

Measuring

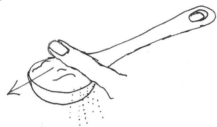

Note: When using measuring spoons, always scoop up the ingredient and run your forefinger over the bowl to level it off, as shown. When measuring liquid, put the measuring jug down on a flat surface to read off the amount – don't tip it. Measuring is very important for gluten-free cooking and baking. It isn't the kind of thing that can be guessed.

Gluten-free apron
Keep a 'dedicated' apron to wear in the kitchen and just keep it for when you are making gluten-free food. This way you can avoid contamination.

Gluten-free lists
Regarding lists of gluten-free foods, you can buy these in the form of a small book. Most of the items listed would probably come into the junk food category.

The list needs to be updated regularly as formulas change and manufacturers stop making certain products or release new ones on to the market all the time.

Supermarket customer services can be contacted for information and there's always the internet, allergy groups and other people who are coping with a gluten-free diet local to you. Ask at the office of your GP surgery for details of any local groups.

I have known of people who spend hours every week reading food labels in supermarkets and others who spend a few hours every week cooking gluten-free. The latter seem to have the better quality of life, better food and better value for money. It is a good idea to keep **your own** little book of gluten-free foods for when you go shopping. A pocket or handbag size notebook with an index is ideal. Names and details of products, shops (telephone nos.) and addresses will come in useful. Keep it up to date as it is important.

This is just a quick glance at the gluten-free problem. It may seem like a very high mountain to climb when you start to try and cope with it but, believe me, you will get used to it because you must.

Always check the label even if it is a product you have used many times before. The manufacturer can change his formula at any time.

Now some technical information to help you understand how things work.

Raising agents

If you were to mix flour and liquid into a heavy paste and bake it in the oven the result would be like a brick – heavy, hard and impossible to chew. If you had mixed a *raising agent* into it the result would have been very different. It would have been lighter and softer.

If a liquid is added to a mixture containing bicarbonate of soda (an alkaline substance), the baking will rise up. However it may well have an unpleasant taste if it isn't neutralized with something acidic. The substance most used for neutralizing is cream of tartar but there are other ingredients that will do the job – yoghurt, milk, golden syrup and lemon juice. Bicarbonate of soda is sometimes used without a neutralizer when a strong flavouring such as ginger has been used. Baking powder has both bicarbonate of soda and cream of tartar in it.

It also has a filler in it to make it keep dry – usually wheat flour. Gluten-free baking powder needs to have a gluten-free filler such as rice flour. Buy from the 'free-from' shelves in a supermarket or at a health store.

How does baking powder work?

Bicarbonate of soda plus cream of tartar and liquid will produce carbon dioxide in cake mixtures. The heat of the oven makes the gas bubbles expand and this gives the lighter texture we expect in cakes. Only relatively small amounts of baking powder are required. Too much will result in a mound of crumbs which will collapse. Baking powder is important and should not be left out if it is given in the recipe or the result will be heavy and flat.

Yeast – how does it work?

Yeast is quite different from baking powder although it can aereate dough to encourage bread rise and make it lighter. Too much yeast will give too great a rise, make the dough weak and spongy with large holes and give the baking a musty taste. It is a greyish/ beige colour and needs to be fed a little sugar to get going (ferment). In bread, given the right warm conditions, it will grow and make the dough double in size. (This is called 'proving'). However, double the rise is the maximum required for a good end product. What will stop it rising is the heat of the oven, during baking. If left in a warm place to rise for too long, so that dough becomes much too light and spongy, all is not lost as it can be 'knocked down', back to its original size and left to rise again. Yeast is traditionally used for bread, rolls, breadsticks, yeasted buns and baking. Baking with yeast can give the bread a crisp crust but a soft inside.

Yeast, you would think is just yeast, but some have additives (not always gluten-free, alas) to make it work more effectively. *When buying yeast, always check the label.* Find a brand which is gluten-free at the supermarket or health store. Once opened it must be re-sealed and stored in the fridge. If you don't re-seal it, it gives up, won't work and dies. Sachets are an expensive way to buy yeast. A little drum or box is much cheaper. Use a clean, dry teaspoon to take from it. Small drums with a plastic lid are easiest to use. Make sure you always keep one in stock.

The recipes in this book use **fast action/instant yeast**, It looks like tiny greyish crumbs. Do not confuse with *dried* active yeast, which looks like grey, hard miniature balls, as they are sold in similar containers. 'Dried' is the key word not 'fast'. It means the yeast has to be soaked in warm water, fed with sugar and encouraged to make froth to show it will work. All this is avoided with *fast action/instant yeast* as it is mixed in dry with other dry ingredients and saves 20 minutes waiting for it to get going.

Storecupboard/fridge/freezer

It is always useful to have a few staples in stock at home for a gluten-free diet.

Two very useful foods are cooked, boiled rice and cooked boiled potatoes which can be stored in the fridge for up to 3 days, covered. Find a suitable gluten-free breakfast cereal and baked beans, cans of sardines and tuna in oil, salmon in brine, eggs, bananas, potatoes and rice, jam, honey, sugar, tea, coffee, milk, cocoa.

Special ingredients are potato flour, cornflour (maize), rice flour, gram flour, Xanthan gum, jam sugar with pectin, gluten-free baking powder and fast action yeast. If you have all these and a supply of fresh/frozen fruit and vegetables, meat and fish, margarine/butter and milk you'll have the basis of a gluten-free diet you can build on.

The next chapter gives you a whole range of gluten-free baking to fill the basic gaps left by not being able to eat gluten. I hope you will see it is not at all difficult.

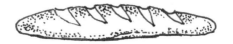

CHAPTER 3

Bread, Basics, Staples

There is more to bread than a loaf from the supermarket shelf or out of the automatic breadmaker. Bread has a history. Early forms of bread were baked in the hearth of the open fire, on a bakestone. Before there were ovens, a cauldron was turned upside down on the bakestone to make a mini oven for baking a loaf. Today we have the equivalent of these in every kitchen and can therefore still make the early forms of bread – scones from the oven or griddle (girdle). As crops became better managed and the gluten content of wheat increased, shaped breads became possible in bakers' ovens. Now we all have ovens at home and can make our own if we wish. We also have hobs on which to make pancakes and pasta. All these foods have something in common – they are made from wheat. It is these that we need to replicate for a gluten-free diet.

So what is so special about wheat? It is known in farming as 'the king of crops', the premier grain, and can be stored after harvest for a long time before being made into bread and a whole range of bakery products. In a healthy Western style diet, wheat accounts for about one fifth of food eaten. In a poor, modern diet much more than that is eaten on account of breakfast cereals, takeaway food, cake, buns, biscuits, snacks, pizzas etc.

This chapter gives you a series of recipes for the basic gluten-free items required for a gluten-free diet – the staples. These will open many doors in the rest of the book. If you are just starting to cook I suggest a good introduction would be to make the early forms of bread, which are very easy. Try dropscones, oven scones and pancakes first, then the soda bread. Those of you who have had experience of cooking and baking with wheat for years will need to try and adjust and take a new style of cooking and baking on board.

All the recipes in this book have been baked or cooked by me personally, with an ordinary domestic stove. My own kitchen is not full of electric tools so please don't feel it is going to be difficult. I have no battery of expensive gadgets and am without staff to help or wash up!

NEW GLUTEN-FREE FLOUR BLEND

Specially for this book, I have designed (formulated) a new gluten-free flour blend. I have called it **'RG77 gluten-free flour blend'** and you will find it in quite a few of the recipes. It is not rocket science and very easy to make. The main difficulty will be getting a supply of the raw materials – rice flour, cornflour (maize), gram (chickpea flour) and potato flour. See chapter 2 for shopping advice. Here is the formula, for the small amount of 8 oz (¼ kilo).

RG77 gluten-free flour blend

2 oz (50g) rice flour,
2 oz (50g) cornflour (maize)
2 oz (50g) potato flour
1 oz (25g) gram flour

It doesn't look very much written down but it does take a long
time and a great deal of experimenting to produce such a formula and work out all the recipes for its use. It is not available
in shops. It is a gluten-free blend for you to make easily at
home.

The method of making the blend is quite simple. Put the 4
flours into a large bowl. Extend the fingers of one hand and
curve them over to make a kind of claw. Mix the flours one
way a few times in a circle, then the other way a few times.
What you are trying to achieve is an even blend. Do this for
a couple of minutes. Use a spoon to transfer to a plastic bag,
seal (I use a clothes peg) and label it with its name and the
date. Now you can begin.

If you get on well with this blend and you need a larger
supply, here are the amounts for a larger amount of it.

RG77 gluten-free flour blend to make 1 lb 5oz (568g)

6 oz (150g) rice flour
6 oz (150g) cornflour (maize)
6 oz (150g) potato flour
3 oz (75g) of gram flour

**Store in a large jar, tin or airtight container in a cool, dry
place – not the fridge. Name and date it.**
The formula is sensitive so it won't work in the recipes if you
leave out one of the ingredients. For cakes, gluten-free baking
powder is added in the recipes. See notes in chapter 2. The
blend can also be used with bicarbonate of soda, cream of
tartar and Xanthan gum.

NO GUESSING!

Please weigh everything out as stated in the recipes. Gluten-

free cooking and baking is not the same as wheat cooking and baking – it is not something that can be guessed. You need to be precise to avoid expensive, disappointing and even inedible baking disasters. Also, the recipes in this book are unlikely to work with a different gluten-free blend. (I can no do more than alert you to this.)

Xanthan Gum
A few words about Xanthan gum. This is not the only binder available but it seems to be quite easy to come by both in health stores and 'free-from' shelves.

It is the 'super-glue' of gluten-free baking that helps to replace gluten, is used in very small quantities and needs care. If you use too much it will make the baking hard and even impossible to bite or chew. However, used in the correct amounts, usually by the pinch, it is an amazing ingredient. If you should spill any on the worktop don't attack it with a wet cloth as it will turn to a shiny film, almost like varnish to look at. It will slither all over your hands and it will be difficult to remove. (I speak from experience.)

See chapter 13 for information on star ratings.

Breakfast dropscones (makes 5) *****
A quickly made substitute for wheat bread.

2 oz (50g) RG77 gluten-free flour blend
1 pinch Xanthan gum
¼ teaspoon cream of tartar
3 pinches bicarbonate of soda
1 pinch salt
½ level teaspoon caster sugar
½ a beaten egg
5 tablespoons milk

1 teaspoon sunflower oil
more sunflower oil for greasing

Method: Mix the flour, Xanthan gum, cream of tartar, bicarbonate of soda, salt and sugar in a bowl. Add the egg and about half the milk. Mix to a thick batter. Beat in the oil and remaining milk to make a smooth batter. Heat a griddle or heavy-based frying pan. Grease lightly and drop tablespoons of the batter on to it, leaving space for them to spread. Cook over a medium heat for a minute until the tops have gone into little holes. Use a palette knife to flip them over to cook on the other side for a minute. They should be golden brown underneath. Keep warm wrapped in a clean tea towel, in a small basket or on a warm plate. Serve instead of wheat bread to spread with margarine or butter.

Teatime dropscones ****
Make as for breakfast dropscones but increase the sugar to 2 teaspoons.

Canapé bases *****
Make the breakfast dropscone batter. Cook in the same way but make small ones by using a teaspoon of batter for each one. They will cook very quickly so leave them on the griddle for less time and don't try and do too many at once. Chapter 12 has details of how to dress them up for a party.

Girdle scones (Farls) – makes 8 very simple and quickly made wedges of bread, on the hob instead of in the oven. If you don't have a griddle a heavy-based frying pan will do just as well. *****

4 oz (100g) RG77 gluten-free flour blend
2 good pinches salt

½ level teaspoon gluten-free baking powder
1 oz (50g) soft margarine
½ oz (15g) caster sugar
1 tablespoon dried milk powder
1 teaspoon fresh lemon juice
3 tablespoons cold water
rice flour for kneading and rolling out
sunflower oil for greasing

Method: Mix the flour, salt and baking powder in a bowl. Rub in the margarine with the fingertips until the mixture resembles breadcrumbs. Stir in the sugar and dried milk. Sprinkle in the lemon juice and spoon in the water. Lightly mix by hand to make a soft dough. Put the griddle or pan on to heat. Dust the worktop with rice flour and shape the dough into a ball. Flatten with your palm and then roll out, using more rice flour, into a round about ½ inch (1 cm) thick. Use a long knife to cut into 8 wedges. Lightly grease the girdle or pan with a screw of kitchen paper and a little sunflower oil. Lower the heat and use a spatula to place the scones on it for about 3 minutes or until brown underneath. They will have puffed up a little. Turn over and cook for 3 minutes on the other side. When they are done they will sound hollow when tapped. Eat freshly baked or on the day of baking, instead of wheat bread.

Oven scones (makes 4 medium,) quickly- made scones ****
These are not the same as tea-time scones as they have no sugar in them. A substitute for bread to eat split and buttered.

4 pinches Xanthan gum
5 oz (140 g) RG77 gluten-free flour blend
2 level teaspoons gluten-free baking powder
pinch salt

1 oz (25g) polyunsaturated soft margarine
1 medium egg, beaten
1 level tablespoon dried milk powder mixed with 1
   tablespoon water

Method: Preheat oven at Gas 7/220° C/425° F. Grease a
baking sheet. Mix the Xantham gum, flour, baking powder
and salt in a bowl. Rub in the margarine until the mixture
resembles crumbs. Work in the egg and milk with a metal
spoon to make a soft, sticky dough. Using a little more of the
flour, knead by hand for a minute. Pat into a ½ inch (1cm)
thick round and cut into quarters. Place apart on the prepared
baking sheet, and bake on the top shelf for about 10-12 minutes, until risen and starting to turn light brown. (Don't brown
them too much or they will be dry.) Cool on a wire rack. Eat
freshly made, split and buttered.

Tea-time scones (makes about 8) small scones ***
Make as for oven scones but add 1 teaspoon caster sugar to
the flour.

Soda bread (makes an 8 oz (225)g round loaf) ****
A quickly made bread for eating as soon as it is baked. It
doesn't keep but can be toasted the next day.

4 oz (125g) RG77 gluten-free flour blend
4 pinches Xanthan gum
¼ level teaspoon bicarbonate of soda
pinch salt
½ oz (15g) polyunsaturated soft margarine
4 tablespoons milk
2 level tablespoons unflavoured yoghurt
4 tablespoons milk
more RG77 flour for kneading

Method: Preheat oven at Gas 7/220° C/425 °F. Mix the flour, Xanthan gum, bicarbonate of soda and salt in a bowl. Rub in the margarine with the fingertips. Put the milk and yoghurt into a basin and whisk with a fork. Make a well in the flour mixture and pour in the milk/yoghurt. Mix together by hand to make a soft dough. Knead for half a minute using more of the flour and shape by hand into a round, about 1 inch (2.5cm) thick. Place on a lightly floured baking tray or a sponge tin and cut a deep cross on the top. Put quickly in the oven on a shelf above centre and bake for about 20 minutes until well risen and the cross has opened up. Take it out of the oven and tap the base. If it sounds hollow, it is done. If not, put back in the oven for a few minutes longer. Leave to cool a little on a wire rack. Serve right away.

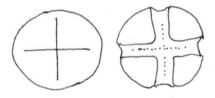

(The roots of soda bread are in Ireland. Folklore has it, the cross opens up to let out the devil. Bearing in mind Ireland now has quite a high rate of its population on a gluten-free diet, maybe folklore has a point.)

BREAD WITH YEAST – THE EVERYDAY LOAF

Bread! What does it mean to most people? Unfortunately the average wheaten loaf has become a squashy, damp sort of sliced cake, with a rubbery crust, a lot of salt, all kinds of additions to make it keep, sliced, wrapped in a plastic bag and made specially to be sold off the supermarket shelf with a shelf-life of several weeks. It is generally bland and with very little taste. It bears little comparison with real bread.

Homemade, handmade wheat bread usually has a crisp crust

with a firmish centre and it smells gorgeous. For people who are able to eat it, it is one of the simple joys of life. Artisan bakers get up at three in the morning to bake in the old way and produce a range of good bread for eating fresh but they are few and far between. All over the country the ping of automatic breadmakers sound, turning out mechanical and electrical uniform loaves, not much different from supermarket fare but nothing like as varied and exciting as old fashioned handmade bread.

Trying to replace wheat bread with gluten-free bread needs a selection of gluten-free flours and several choices of binder to replace the lost gluten, the wheat protein that enables shaped breads to be made. Without gluten, that magical protein in wheat, bread just collapses into a heap of crumbs, as it is the gluten that binds it all together.

Designing new kinds of bread made without the gluten flours wheat, rye, barley or possibly oats requires regard to the following:

Appearance – Does it look like bread? Does it look appetizing? Does it look like what it is supposed to?
Taste – Does it taste like bread or is it a disappointment? Does it have a good aftertaste?
Texture – Is there a marked difference between the crust and the centre? Is the crust crisp? Is the centre firm but chewable?
Colour – Does the colour look right?
Aroma – Does it smell like bread? Does it make you want to eat it?
Nutrition – Is it nourishing? Does it have enough protein or is it just mainly starch? Is it a good food or is it just gluten-free junk food?
Ease of making – can it be made easily without a lot of expensive gadgets?
Appeal – Is it enviable or is it a food that will make people feel sorry for you?

Digestible quality – Is it easy to digest?
Ingredients – Are the ingredients easy to obtain?
Price – Are the ingredients a reasonable price?

This might seem to be a design nightmare but it all has to be borne in mind when designing a new kind of bread without gluten. What also has to be considered is that bread doesn't just mean loaves of bread. Rolls and scones, pancakes, pasta, pastry, biscuits, cakes, pastries, noodles etc. are all kinds of bread. The task is enormous.

There was a time when men in white coats in laboratories did the designing. (The results were not inspiring or a pleasure to eat.) Since then women have put on their aprons and got to work in the kitchen at home. Now the situation is much more exciting and gluten-free food much better with a greater understanding of what the gluten-free dieter wants to eat.

If you are used to baking wheat loaves, put that knowledge out of your head. Here is a gluten-free loaf that is mixed up like a batter and put straight into the oven on a low heat. Here it rises, cracks open and allows the top half to form. It is crusty, smells like bread, and looks and tastes like bread. It is not an exact replica of wheat bread but it is nutritious and very quick and easy to make.

The recipe is for a small loaf and does not multiply up to make a larger loaf in a larger tin. If you want more than this in one go, make more than one loaf the same size.

(Experienced wheat bakers are inclined not to believe this loaf is possible. I can assure you it is.)

Quick Gluten-free Loaf – makes 1 small, golden loaf with a good flavour and aftertaste. Eat freshly baked, for sandwiches, fried bread, toast, breadcrumbs, stuffing and bread sauce. An all round gluten-free loaf of bread. The binder is egg. No need to let it rise before baking as it will do this in the oven. To make lukewarm water put 1 cup hot water from the kettle into a jug with 2 cups of cold. Stir and use immediately before it cools. (Do not use an electric blender or beaters to make the loaf instead of a wooden spoon as they are too fierce. They will only make the bread tough.) ****

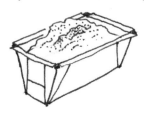

7g fast action instant yeast (1 slightly heaped teaspoon)
4½ oz (115g) potato flour
1 oz (25g) gram flour
3 oz (75g) cornflour (maize)
¾ oz (20g) ground almonds
1 level teaspoon caster sugar
2 good pinches salt
1 medium egg, whisked in a cup
¼ pint (150ml) lukewarm water, minus 1 tablespoon

Method: Preheat oven at Gas 4/180° C/350° F. Carefully grease an old-fashioned 1lb (500g) loaf tin with margarine, making sure you get into the corners. Put the dry ingredients into a bowl and mix well. Stir in the egg and water. Pour into the flour mixture. Use a wooden spoon to mix then beat to a smooth batter. Turn into the prepared tin and bake above centre shelf for about 50 minutes. Test with a skewer while still in the tin. If it comes out clean the loaf is done. If it doesn't, put it back into the oven for another 5 minutes and test again. Turn out carefully on to a wire rack to cool. Use when cold to prevent cracking. (The loaf needs to rest.) Store wrapped in a plastic bag, sealed. Eat within 3 days, freshly made or toasted.

It can be frozen on the day of baking. Defrost slowly before using.

White Dough for Shaped Breads, Rolls, Breadsticks, Baps and Pizza bases makes 10 oz (280 g) of dough).
Enough for 4 large or 6 small rolls or a shaped loaf

2 oz (50g) cornflour (maize)
3 oz (75g) potato flour
½ oz (15g) ground almonds
¼ teaspoon salt
¼ level teaspoon + 2 pinches Xanthan gum
1 level teaspoon caster sugar
2 level teaspoons died milk powder
1 level teaspoon fast action instant yeast
1 medium egg beaten with 4 tablespoons lukewarm water
more potato flour for kneading etc.

This is the basic dough for shaped breads

Baps (makes 4) ****
Use the white dough ingredients as above.

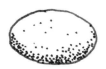

Method: Grease a baking sheet. Put the first seven ingredients into a bowl. Mix well for a minute with both hands to make sure they are evenly distributed. Sprinkle in the yeast and mix again. Make a well in the centre and add the egg/water. Mix with a metal spoon to make 1 ball of dough. Dust the worktop with potato flour and turn out the dough on to it. Knead for 1 minute until you a have a smooth elastic dough. (You can do this with one hand.) Make into 1 ball and divide into 4 quarters. Shape into baps and put on to the baking sheet. Slash with a knife (see suggestions) and loosely cover with food film and a clean tea towel. Leave to rise in a warm place until doubled in size and puffed up. Bake in a preheated oven at Gas 7/220° C/425° F on the top shelf for 15 minutes until golden and crisp. Eat freshly baked. Any left over can be frozen when cold. They need to thaw slowly and be baked in the oven for 5 minutes to re-crisp them.

French Stick (baton) – a shaped loaf ****

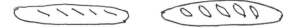

Make the dough as for baps but use a large egg and keep 2 teaspoons of the beaten egg back, on a saucer. Make the French stick into a long sausage and put diagonally on a greased baking sheet. Brush with the egg from the saucer. Slash diagonally with a sharp knife – this helps it to rise. Leave to rise in a warm place, covered with a piece of food film and a clean tea towel. When it has doubled in size and the slashes have opened, bake on the top shelf for about 15 minutes. Eat freshly baked.

Shaped Rolls (makes 6) ****
Make the dough as for baps and roll into a long sausage. Cut in half then cut each piece into 3 to give you 6. The dough is quite elastic and can be shaped into a round, knot, mini bloomer, coil or plait, using more of the potato flour. Brush with milk or egg and water and sprinkle with poppy seeds or sesame seeds.

Slash the mini-bloomer diagonally, the round rolls with a

cross or as shown in the diagram. You can also snip with kitchen scissors in a pattern. To make the plait, roll into a long thin sausage and divide into three. Pinch 3 together and plait loosely. Pinch the 3 ends together. They will all neaten up in the rising. When doubled in size and looking puffy, bake on the top shelf as for baps.

Eat freshly baked and crisp.

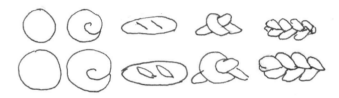

Coburg (makes 1 small round loaf) with a characteristic top.
****

Make the dough as for baps and shape into a round, domed loaf. After you have placed in a greased sponge tin, brush with milk and sprinkle with poppy seeds. Slash the top to make shapes as shown in the diagram. Cover with food film and a clean tea towel. Leave to rise in a warm place. When

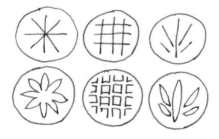

doubled in size and the slashes have opened up to make the chosen pattern, bake in a preheated oven at Gas 6/200°C/400° F, above centre shelf for about 25 – 30 minutes. To see if the loaf is done, turn it upside down and tap the base. Does it sound hollow? If it does, it is baked. Cool on a wire rack. As soon as it is cold, wrap in food film. Eat freshly baked. Toast the following day.

Flavoured Breads all ****
The white dough will take additions. Work them in when you knead. Choose one from the following:

- 1 tablespoon of chopped sun-dried **tomato**
- 5 destoned, chopped, plain, black or green **olives**
- 4 **walnut** halves, finely chopped (but not ground)
- 1 heaped teaspoon finely chopped fresh, **mixed herbs**
- ½ clove **garlic** put through a crusher

Foccacia – olive oil bread ***
Make the white dough as for baps. Grease a sponge tin and put the dough in the centre. Press out with the fingers to make a flat, round shape about ½ an inch (1.25cm) thick. Poke a finger in all over. Drizzle with a little olive oil so it goes into the dents and scatter with sea salt and a few sprigs of fresh

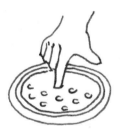

rosemary. Cover with food film and a clean tea towel. Leave to rise and double in size in a warm place. Bake on the top shelf of the oven at Gas 7/220° C/425° F for about 15 minutes. Cut into wedges and take out of the tin. Serve still warm from the oven.

Pizza bases

Bread based pizza ****
The white dough for shaped bread is ideal for a pizza with a true bread base. When you have made the dough, press out thinly on a greased baking sheet and roll over it with a rolling pin. Pinch up an edge all the way round to contain the filling. Preheat oven at Gas 7/220°C/425° F. Top the pizza as suggested in chapter 7, cover with food film and leave it to rise in a warm place until the base looks puffy. (If you are in a hurry put it straight into the oven.) Bake for about 15 minutes (or less) on the top shelf. The amount of dough in the recipe will make 2 large (dinner size) or 4 small (snack size). Use what you need and make the rest of the dough into rolls.

Scone based pizza ****
For a pizza with a **scone base** use the dough from the **oven scones** recipe in the same way but don't leave it to rise – arrange the topping and put it straight into the oven, preheated at Gas 7/220°C/425° F, on the top shelf. It doesn't matter which type of base you use as both are kinds of bread. Obviously, the scone base is quicker to make because it only needs to rise during baking and not before.

Breadsticks ****
Roll out the white dough for shaped bread, thinly, on a sheet of baking parchment, floured with potato flour. Use a sharp knife to cut into long strings. Roll each one using both hands into a long, thin sausage. Place on a greased baking sheet. Cover with food film and leave to rise in a warm place. When doubled in size, bake at the top of the oven, preheated at Gas 7/220 °C/425° F for 5 minutes or longer until pale gold. Cool on a wire rack. Wrap in food film. Best eaten on the day of baking.
   Note: Short versions are easier to handle.

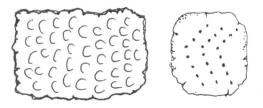

Crispbreads (makes 4 large) *****

 1 oz (25g) rice flour
 1 oz (25g) potato flour
 ½ oz (15g) gram flour
 2 pinches sugar
 4 pinches salt
 2 pinches Xanthan gum
 2 tablespoons sunflower oil
 2 tablespoons cold water
 2 tablespoons finely grated cooking apple (or plain stewed
    apple)

Method: Preheat oven at Gas 7/220° C/425 °F. Line a baking
sheet with baking parchment. Mix the six dry ingredients in
a bowl. Add the oil and rub in with the fingertips until it
resembles crumbs. Put in the water and apple and mix by
hand to a stiff dough. Put on to the prepared baking sheet and
press out with the fingers. Roll out with a rolling pin and press
all over with two fingertips to make a coarse, dimpled, crisp-
bready texture. Cut into four (or 8) and bake on the top shelf
for about 15 minutes until golden.

   Put on to a wire rack to cool. Store wrapped in food film,
in an airtight container. These will keep well but are nicest
freshly baked. For a better flavour use margarine instead of
the oil.

Seeded crispbreads (makes 4 large or 8 small) *****
Omit the texturing with the fingertips and leave flat. Brush
with either beaten egg white, milk or water and sprinkle with
sesame seeds or poppy seeds. For a multi-seed crispbread,
make as for seeded but use linseeds, sunflower seeds, sesame
and poppy seeds, mixed. Press them into the crispbread and
use more than a sprinkle.

Crispbread with nuts and seeds *****
Make as for seeded crispbreads but add nuts as well as the
seeds – finely chopped almonds, walnuts, cashews etc. Avoid
commercial nut mixes as they are usually heavy on peanuts
and light on proper nuts.

Crispbreads with rice bran (makes 10) *****

1½ oz (40g) rice flour
½ oz (15g) cornflour
½ oz (15g) gram flour
2 pinches salt
3 pinches caster sugar
½ level tablespoon rice bran
¾ oz (20g) polyunsaturated soft margarine
1 oz (25g) mashed potato (fresh)
2 tablespoons water

Method: Preheat oven at Gas 7/ 220 °C/425° F. Put the first
6 dry ingredients into a bowl and mix well to combine. Add
the margarine and rub in until the mixture resembles crumbs.
Stir in the potato with a fork and then put in the water. Work
together by hand. Keep going and don't add any more water.
Make into 1 very stiff lump. Dust the worktop with a little rice
flour and form the dough into a sausage. Cut off 10 equal
slices. Roll out each one into an oval about 3 in (7cm) long

and place on a baking sheet lined with baking parchment. Use a fork to prick each one in a pattern and make them all the same. Bake for 10 minutes on the top shelf, then turn them over for another 3 minutes. Cool on a wire rack. When cold, wrap individually or in food film and store in an airtight container. These will keep well, like ordinary crispbreads. Try the health store for rice bran.

Crackers (makes 10) ****
These are plain biscuits to eat with cheese.

   2 oz (50g) RG77 gluten-free flour blend
   3 pinches salt
   1 pinch caster sugar
   1 small pinch Xanthan gum (optional)
   ½ oz (15g) polyunsaturated soft margarine
   2 tablespoons cold water
   rice flour

Method: Preheat oven at Gas 7/225° C/425°F. Cut a sheet of baking parchment to fit a baking tray. Put the flour into a bowl with the salt, sugar and Xanthan gum. Mix well. Rub in the margarine with the fingers until the mixture resembles crumbs. Add 2 tablespoons (exactly, don't guess) cold water. Mix by hand to make a sticky paste. Add a little rice flour and work it in to make a stiffer, less sticky paste. Knead for 30 seconds to make it smooth, using more rice flour. Dust the baking parchment with rice flour and roll out the dough thinly. Cut into squares with a sharp knife to make 10 crackers. Make holes right through with the point of the knife, in a pattern. (Do the same on each one). Put the baking parchment with the crackers on to the baking tray and bake on the top shelf for 10 minutes. Turn the biscuits over and bake for another 3 minutes until the edges begin to turn golden. Cool on a wire rack – they will crisp up as they cool. When cold, wrap individually in food film and store in an airtight container.

Choux Pastry
Choux pastry is the thinnest pastry, meant to bake into edible casings for éclairs, profiteroles and buns filled with cream. (Party food, not everyday food.)

Basic Choux Pastry (enough for 10 profiteroles or 5 eclairs)
****

3 tablespoons cold water
3 pinches caster sugar
½ oz (15g) polyunsaturated soft margarine
2 teaspoons sunflower oil
1½ oz (40g) RG77 gluten-free flour blend
1 medium egg, beaten

Method: Preheat oven at Gas 6/200° C/400° F Put the water, sugar, margarine and oil into a medium saucepan. Heat gently until the margarine has melted. Tip in the flour, all in one go, and stir over a medium heat until it forms one ball of dough. Take off the heat and gradually beat in the egg. Beat to a smooth stiff paste. Use a teaspoon to break off lumps of dough into the size and number you require. Wet your hands in cold water and shape the lumps into balls or 'sausages', putting them on to a greased baking sheet, floured with rice flour. The water will make the shapes smooth and they will rise during baking. (If you prefer them textured, leave them as they are.) Bake for 20 – 25 minutes, depending on size. When the pastries are baked they will be crisp and golden. You will need to slit each one open with a knife.

Use a teaspoon to carefully remove any uncooked dough left inside. Put back into the oven for another 5 minutes to dry them

on the inside. Cool on a wire rack and use on the day of baking.
Use the slit to put in the filling. Use the dough as directed in the
recipes for profiteroles, éclairs and choux buns in chapter 3.
Make fresh when you need to use it. See chapter 12 for
Celebration food recipes.

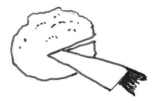

Yorkshire Puddings I (makes 6 small, enough for 2 portions)
****

Make as for basic choux pastry but omit sugar and add 1 good
pinch salt. Divide into 6 and shape into balls. Put on a greased
baking sheet floured with rice flour. Bake on the centre shelf
at Gas 6/200° C/400° F, until well risen and golden. Take out
of the oven and cut a slit in each one with a knife. If you find
too much uncooked dough inside them, remove with a teaspoon via the slit. Crisp and golden, these small 'Yorkshires'
can be made well ahead of a roast dinner for the gluten-free
dieter and warmed as required.

Yorkshire Puddings II (makes 4) *****

These are made with a batter in the traditional way and can be
served to everyone. They are easier to make than wheat
Yorkshires as the flour doesn't tend to go into lumps. Because
there is no gluten in them, they should fall out of the tin
instead of getting stuck – good news for the cook. You will
need the traditional, four-pan Yorkshire pudding tin.

1 oz (25g) RG77 gluten-free flour blend
1 pinch gluten-free baking powder

1 pinch salt
1 medium egg
2 tablespoons milk
3 tablespoons cold water

Method: Put the flour into a basin with the baking powder and salt. Mix. Add the egg and stir in until you have a lump-free, thick paste. Spoon in the milk and water and mix/beat to a thin batter. Oil a 4 x pan Yorkshire pudding tin with sunflower oil and a screw of kitchen paper. Heat up on the hob or in a hot oven. Use a small jug to pour the batter equally into the pans. Bake at the top of a hot oven for about 15 -20 minutes or longer, until well risen and crisp. Turn them over and continue cooking for another 5 minutes. Keep warm in the bottom of the oven.

Note: Batter can be used immediately or allowed to stand for a while, until required.

PASTRY

In the early days of pastry, centuries ago, pastry was more like a biscuit, made from flour and water. It was not meant to be eaten but to contain semi-liquid food while it cooked e.g. a stew. (They were called coffins.) These containers, along with hard baked trenchers used by the rich as large plates, were given to the grateful poor, who did eat them. They were popular as they were not only free but tasty too. The pastry we know today springs from these. Pastry now contains fat and is intended for consumption, along with the food it contains. It is a cross between bread and biscuit. Sometimes it is baked 'blind', meaning empty, to be filled after baking. Commercially-made wheat-gluten pastry can often resemble cardboard and is not something to be emulated. A good shortcrust pastry should be a little crisp on the bite and crumbly in the mouth.

Gluten-free shortcust pastry causes a dilemma. If there is enough binder in it to make the raw dough elastic, the baked result will be too hard and difficult to bite and chew, although it will look perfect. The following pastry does not have a binder.

Shortcrust pastry (makes just over 4 oz (100g)) ***
Enough for 4 tartlets with lids or 6 tartlet cases to bake blind. It will make 1 pie lid, a case for tarte du jour or 1 medium/2 small pasties.

1½ oz (40g) rice flour
1½ oz (40g) potato flour
1 heaped teaspoon ground almonds
2 good pinches salt
2 pinches caster sugar
1¼ oz (30g) polyunsaturated margarine
½ tablespoons cold water
more rice flour for kneading etc.

Method: Put the rice flour, potato flour, ground almonds, salt and sugar into a bowl and mix well to distribute evenly. Add the margarine and rub in with the fingertips until the mixture resembles crumbs. Measure in the water (don't guess) and mix by hand to a stiff paste. Use a little rice flour to knead for a few seconds until smooth. Roll out on a piece of baking parchment, using very little rice flour.

The recipes in chapters 7, 9, 10 and 12 will tell you how to use this pastry for pies, tarts, savoury straws etc.

Shortcrust pastry top for a pie ***
Have your pie filling *ready cooked.* Roll out the shortcrust pastry in a circle, on a sheet of baking parchment, slightly larger than the pie. Cut off a narrow piece all the way round

with a sharp knife and use in pieces to line the wetted edge of the pie dish, mending as you go. Brush with cold water. Fill the pie dish with your chosen filling. Move the pastry lid to the pie, turn it upside down and place on the pie. Peel off the baking parchment. Press the edge down all the way round and trim with a knife to neaten. Press all round with the tines of a fork or pinch between finger and thumb. Cut a hole in the centre to let out the steam. Bake for about 15 minutes in a pre-heated oven at Gas 7/220° C/425° F, near the top of the oven. A savoury pie can be brushed with a little beaten egg to give a shiny golden finish.

If you feel this is too difficult, just bake the pastry in a circle, with a pinched up edge, still on the baking parchment. Cut in wedges and serve on top of the cooked filling. Easy!

Apple pastry (for steaming) ****
Use this as a substitute for suet pastry and you have a wheat-free and gluten-free pastry you can serve to the whole family. It will line a 1 pint (600ml) pudding basin and give enough to make a lid.

2 oz (50g) suitable soft margarine
4 oz (110g) ground rice
3 oz (75g) finely grated eating apple

Method: Put the ingredients into a bowl and blend with a fork. Knead by hand into a ball of stiff paste, adding a little more ground rice if required. Put two thirds into the basin and press out with the fingers to line it. Use the remaining pastry for the lid. For the filling us plums, apricots, apple etc. Cover and steam in the usual way. See chapter 9.

Egg pasta (makes 2 portions for tagliatelle, ravioli and lasagna) ****

4 oz (100g) RG77 gluten-free flour blend
1 large egg
2 teaspoons extra virgin olive oil
¼ teaspoon salt
1 tablespoon water
more RG77 flour or rice flour for kneading and rolling out

Method: Put on a medium pan of water to boil. Put the flour into a bowl and make a well in the centre. Mix the egg, oil and salt in a basin and pour into the well. Use your fingers to mix into large pieces. Sprinkle in the water and work into 1 ball of dough. Flour the worktop and using more of the flour, knead the dough for 2 or 3 minutes. If it is too sticky, add a little more of the flour. If it is too dry add a little more water. The dough should be smooth and a little elastic. Flour the worktop again and roll out with a rolling pin. Without moving it around, roll one way and then the other until the dough is thin. Cut with a pizza wheel or pasta wheel unto thin strands, flat noodles (tagliatelle), squares (for ravioli) or larger oblongs for lasagna. (See note below.) Use a fish slice to take the pasta off the worktop and use quickly, putting it into a pan of boiling water. It should be boiled for 5 – 6 minutes then drained in a colander and put back into the empty but still warm pan. Gently stir in a knob of margarine to coat the hot pasta. (This stops the pasta from sticking together in clumps.) Use right away.

See Chapter 7 for recipes for main meals using pasta – spaghetti Bolognese, ravioli and lasagna.

Note: *Some will find the rolling out easier if done between 2 sheets of food film. Put food film on the worktop making sure you have allowed for the pasta to increase in area. Dust with RG77 flour or rice flour. Flatten out the dough first by hand, then dust with flour. Cover with a sheet of food film. Use the rolling pin on top of this. When you have finished rolling out, carefully peel off the top layer of food film. When you have cut it up, take off the pasta with a fish slice and put it straight into a pan of boiling water.*

Crispy Noodles (1 portion) for Chinese meals and snax (nibbles).See chapters 7 and 4. ***

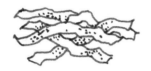

1 oz (25g) RG77 gluten-free flour blend
pinch salt
1½ tablespoons cold water
rice flour for rolling out
sunflower oil for frying

Method: Put the flour and salt into a basin with the water. Mix by hand to a stiff dough. Knead for 1 minute using a little rice flour. Dust a piece of baking parchment with rice flour and roll out the dough thinly. Use a sharp knife or a pizza cutter to cut long strips about two tenths of an inch (½ cm) wide. Heat shallow sunflower oil in a saucepan. Peel off the noodles into the hot oil. Fry for a minute then turn them over and fry for another minute. When they are crisp and, take out of the pan with a slotted spoon and put on to kitchen paper to drain. Leave to grow cold on a plate. Use with Chinese food – see chapter 7.

Snack crispy noodles (snax)
Make as for crispy noodles but cut into short lengths. After frying, sprinkle with a pinch of salt. When cold put into a container or plastic bag. Use within 3 days.

Pancakes (makes 3) ****

2 oz (50g) RG77 gluten-free flour blend
pinch salt
1 egg
¼ pint (150 ml) milk
sunflower oil for greasing pan

Method: Put a plate to warm. Put the flour into a basin with the salt and egg. Mix to a thick paste. Add the milk a little at a time and stir in to make the paste into a thin batter. Pour a little oil into a saucer and use a screw of kitchen paper to grease a frying pan. Put over the heat and when really hot, pour in one third of the batter, tilting the pan to make it run all over the base. Cook for a minute or two then flip over with a spatula to cook on the other side for a minute. Keep warm while you make two more. See chapters 7 and 9 for finishing.

Note: If you don't have any RG77 flour, use 1½ oz (40g) rice flour with ½ oz (15g) cornflour.

Pan Pasta (makes 1 portion) ****
A really quick pasta. Have your sauce ready before you make the pancakes.

Use the pancake batter made with RG77 flour to make 3 pancakes but cook for only 1 minute each side, or less, so that they are soft and not crisp. Roll up and cut off thin slices to make tagliatelle and even thinner slices to make spaghetti. To make pasta for lasagna, cut into rectangles. For other, smaller shapes, cut into squares and triangles. See chapters 7 and 8 for sauces etc.

(This kind of pasta is not suitable for ravioli.)

Chapati (makes 4 medium) *****
Crisp, with a ragged edge and golden blisters. A very ancient and basic kind of bread to serve with curries and salads or as a snack.

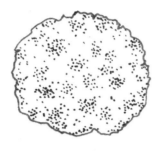

2 oz (50g) RG77 gluten-free flour blend
1 pinch salt
1 pinch Xanthan gum
2 tablespoons water
1 tablespoon sunflower oil
rice flour for rolling out

Method: Put the flour, salt and Xanthan gum into a bowl. Mix well to distribute evenly. Add the water and oil. Use a metal spoon to mix into a sticky lump. Dust the worktop with rice flour. Knead for a minute until the dough is smooth. Form into a ball and cut into 4 equally sized pieces. Roll each piece into a ball and put on to a worktop covered with a piece of food film, floured with rice flour. Flour the dough and put another piece of food film on top. Use a rolling pin, rolling from top to bottom and side to side without moving the chapati between the two layers of food film. Roll out to paper thin. Take off the top piece of food film and gently peel off the chapati. Place in a hot, heavy based, dry frying pan – no need for any oil. Over a medium heat, cook the chapatti for 1 or 2 minutes. The surface will blister. Turn over and cook on the other side for a minute. Use the same food film for the next 3. Stack on a plate. Perfect with curry and rice. Make as required and eat freshly made.

Muffins

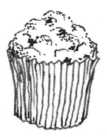

These are not like English muffins, instead, they are a cross between a semi-sweet or savoury bun/bread and a scone – large buns with cracked tops, bursting with fruit etc. The sweet ones contain about 1 oz (25g) of fresh fruit and the savoury ones have all kinds of savoury additions. They are larger than cup cakes and require muffin tins and muffin papers for lining the tins.

The savoury ones can be eaten for breakfast or brunch, snacks or accompaniments to soup, tea and supper The sweet versions are good for a snack or for tea and are popular for lunchboxes and picnics if they are packed in a small container. They are best eaten just as they are without decorations, icing or prettying up. They weigh between 2 and 3 ounces (50 – 75g) so are quite substantial. They are meant to be eaten freshly baked and are not designed to keep.

Fruit muffins (makes 4) ***

  2½ oz (70g) RG77 gluten-free flour blend
  ½ oz (15g) ground almonds
  1 level teaspoon gluten-free baking powder
  1 oz (25g) caster sugar
  2 oz (50g) polyunsaturated soft margarine
  1 medium egg
  fruit and flavouring – see list below

Method: Preheat oven at Gas 6/200° C/400° F. Have ready the fruit and flavouring of your choice. Put the flour, ground almonds, baking powder, sugar, margarine and egg into a bowl. Mix/beat to a smooth cream. Add the fruit and flavouring of your choice and mix in. Divide between the 4 paper cases and bake. They are baked when pressed with a finger they spring back. Leave in the tins for 5 minutes before turning out on to a wire rack to cool. Eat freshly baked, still warm if possible.

***Fruit and flavours*:** Choose one. If using canned fruit buy ones in fruit juice and not syrup. Drain well before using.

- ½ a banana, 4 chopped walnut halves and ½ teaspoon ground cinnamon.
- 2 heaped tablespoons fresh blueberries or raspberries and 4 drops vanilla flavouring.
- 2 heaped tablespoons fresh, chopped strawberries and 4 drops vanilla flavouring.
- 2 heaped tablespoons fresh blackberries, or 1 tablespoon of blackberries and ½ a chopped eating apple.
- 2 ripe dessert plums, destined and chopped.
- ½ a ripe dessert pear chopped and 1 teaspoon cocoa with 3 drops of vanilla flavouring.

- 8 canned apricot halves, chopped.
- 10 fresh cherries, destoned and chopped.
- 1 chopped fresh or canned pineapple ring with 4 drops vanilla flavouring.
- 2 heaped tablespoons fresh or defrosted summerfruits.

Note: It is a good idea to keep back a little of the fruit and press it into the top of the muffins before baking. This way it indicates what fruit has been used.

Savoury muffins (makes 3) ****

2½ oz (65g) RG77 gluten-free flour blend
1 level teaspoon gluten-free baking powder
2 level tablespoons ground almonds
2 pinches salt
¼ teaspoon sugar
2 tablespoons sunflower oil,
1 medium egg, beaten
2 tablespoons milk
savoury additions etc. of your choice – see list below

Method: Preheat oven at Gas 5/220° C/425° F. Line a muffin tin with 3 papers. Put the flour, baking powder, ground almonds, salt and sugar into a bowl. Mix well. Add the oil, egg and milk. Mix to a smooth, very soft dough. Work in the savoury additions of your choice. Divide equally between the muffin cases and bake above centre of the oven for about 20 minutes, until well risen and golden brown. Press with a finger to see if they are done. If the muffin springs back they are done. Leave in the tin for 5 minutes then transfer to a wire rack to cool. Eat still warm from the oven or the same day. For breakfast, brunch, lunch, tea, a snack or supper.

Savoury additions – choose one to weigh 2 – 3 oz (50 -75g) in total.

- ½ stick celery chopped small, 1 heaped tablespoon grated cheddar cheese.
- ham (without breadcrumb coating), spring onion and chopped fried mushrooms.
- 6 chopped pitted black olives, 1 chopped sundried tomato and 1 chopped spring onion.
- lean from 1 rasher of back bacon, fried and cut into small squares with 1 small mushroom chopped and fried (with the bacon).
- finely grated raw courgette, finely grated tasty cheddar cheese and 1 chopped spring onion.
- cheese, ¼ of an eating apple, chopped and 3 ground walnuts.
- finely grated carrot, chopped walnuts and finely chopped onion
- chopped cooked beetroot, a little chopped blue cheese and a chopped spring onion.
- 1 sundried tomato (or 1 small fresh) chopped, 1 spring onion chopped and 3 chopped leaves of basil with ½ a clove of garlic put through a crusher.
- finely chopped red pepper and 3 chopped black olives.

Mini muffin breads (makes 3) *****
Use the recipe for savoury muffins but omit the flavouring and additions. Cut squares of baking parchment.

As they only take 20 minutes to bake they are ideal for breakfast. Get the dry ingredients ready in a mixing bowl the night before, ready to add oil, egg and milk. Have the muffin tin ready with the parchment papers cut. If you give them an extra 3 minutes in the oven you can get a crust on the top.

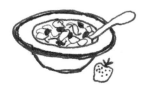

CHAPTER 4

Breakfast, Snacks And Nibbles

This chapter is more about ideas and links to other chapters in the book than specific recipes. Some of the suggestions will seem rather simple and obvious but a few people who will read this book will have no cookery, shopping or gluten-free experience whatsoever.

Breakfast gets its name from 'fast', the overnight lack of food, and 'break' meaning it is the end of the fast. So when we get up in the morning we have had nothing to eat for at least eight hours, perhaps even ten hours or more. Anyone who goes without breakfast is extending that fast to even more hours. Actually, breakfast is an important meal and an essential start to the day.

Most people are in a rush to get to work or school in the mornings and prefer food that is quick to prepare such as breakfast cereal or a quickly cooked egg dish. The breakfast cereal shelves in any supermarket are a minefield for the gluten-free dieter as most of them are based on wheat. Even the non-wheat ones can have gluten added or be contaminated if they are manufactured and packed in factories where wheat is also processed. Many breakfast cereals border on confectionery with high levels of sugar and added chocolate etc. Should *anyone* be eating them? If you prefer a plain commercial breakfast cereal, try to find a brand of cornflakes that is gluten-free. This will be labeled 'gluten-free' and the most likely place to buy them will be a health food store. This is because almost all major brands of cornflakes have what is called a 'barley wash' as part of their manufacture. (Barley is not gluten-free.) Rice based breakfast cereals can be treated in the same way. However, if you look hard enough you will find ones to suit a gluten-free diet. This might mean time spent in the cereal aisles of supermarkets with a magnifying glass, but the quickest answer to this will probably be a swift call to your health food store, or another gluten-free dieter with experience.

HOT BREAFASTS

Breakfasts can be hot or cold. This first one is a hot one, ever popular and naturally gluten-free. It could be described as a gluten-free 'full English'.

Bacon and egg (serves 1) **
Cut the lean from 2 or 3 thin rashers of back bacon and fry gently in 1 tablespoon of sunflower oil. Have ready a warmed plate. When cooked, dab with a double thickeness of kitchen paper to remove excess oil. Keep warm while you fry the egg. Put on to the plate and serve. As this is the bare minimum, consider slices of cold boiled potato, lightly fried at the same time as the bacon, also 1 or 2 halved fresh tomatoes.

Another popular product you might need to search for is a brand of gluten-free baked beans. (Always check each time you use them to make sure the manufacturer has not changed the formula.) Quite a simple task, to assemble this dish, illustrates the lot of the gluten-free dieter. What does an ordinary person do? They go to the supermarket, buy any tin of baked beans and any wheat loaf. The gluten-free dieter, on the other hand, needs special gluten-free bread and a specific brand of gluten-free baked beans. A special diet needs special knowledge.

Beans on toast (serves 1) ***
Toast slices of gluten-free bread and put a plate to warm. Heat a portion of gluten-free baked beans. Spread polyunsaturated soft margarine on the toast and top with the hot beans. Raise the nourishment by putting a poached egg on top.

Bacon and baked beans (serves 1) ***
Bacon doesn't necessarily have to be served with egg. Bacon and fried cold potato and a gluten-free table sauce makes a good breakfast with a piece of fresh fruit. The cold potato can have been boiled or baked. If there isn't any cooked potato available try reheated boiled rice,.

Fishcakes (serves 1) ****
See chapter 7 for this recipe. Shallow fry 2 fishcakes and serve on a warm plate with 2 tablespoons chopped, peeled plum tomatoes, heated through in a small pan with a pinch of salt and 2 pinches sugar. Serve on a warm plate.

Note: If you don't want to do egg and gluten-free breadcrumb coating, just coat the fishcakes with cornflour and fry in shallow fat.

Sausages and tomato ***
Make homemade gluten-free sausages from the recipes in chapter 7, either pork or beef. Serve 2 per person with either

grilled fresh tomatoes or chopped, canned peeled plum tomatoes. Put into a small pan with a pinch of salt and 2 pinches of sugar per person and heat through. Serve on a warm plate.

Smoked haddock and poached egg (serves 1) ****
Poach 1 portion of smoked haddock in milk for 5 minutes or until cooked. Drain. Put on to a warm plate and keep warm while you poach an egg. Put a knob of margarine on top of the fish to melt. Top with the egg and serve with gluten-free bread.

Pancakes (serves 1) ***
See chapter 3 for pancake batter and how to cook them and chapter 9 for filling suggestions. Either fruit or savoury gluten-free pancakes are good for breakfast.

Bubble and squeak (serves 1) ****
This is more of a brunch or late breakfast than an early start. Traditionally this dish is made of leftovers from the previous day's roast dinner. It is useful because it is naturally gluten-free and goes with any kind of meat or eggs.
Put a knob of margarine into a frying pan and melt over a low heat. Add cold boiled potato, chopped and ½ a portion of cooked boiled cabbage, also chopped. Turn them over with a fish slice to mix and turn up the heat to fry. Press the fish slice on the mixture to compress it. Cook for about 2 or 3 minutes then turn over to cook on the other side for another 2 minutes. It should be browned and crispy on both sides. Put on to a cold plate and serve with sliced cold meat such as ham, pork, lamb, or beef off a cold roast joint, chicken etc. A table sauce (see chapter 8) will be welcome. Serve with an omelet or fried egg on a warm plate. See chapter 6 for more details about a variety of ingredients for bubble and squeak.

EGGS (all for 1 serving)
Omelet (see chapter 7)

Poached egg *****
Use a small frying pan. Half fill with boiling water from the kettle. Have ready an egg broken into a cup. Take a fork and stir the hot water round quickly to make a little swirl. Let the egg slide out of the cup into the centre. Bring the pan back to the boil then lower the heat and simmer gently to set the white. Spoon out as much water as you can then lift out the poached egg with a spatula or fish slice. (Avoid tipping the pan to pour out the water as the egg will be very slippery and will likely slide out with the water into the sink.) Serve on gluten-free bread, toasted and spread with margarine.

Scrambled eggs *****
Break 2 eggs into a basin. Add 1 tablespoon suitable milk (or water). Break the yolks with a fork and stir to lightly combine the yolks, transparent white and milk. Pour into a small, lightly greased pan (preferably non-stick) and put over a gentle heat. As the eggs begin to set break them up with a spoon. When almost set but still looking creamy on top, serve hot on gluten-free toast spread with margarine.

Fried egg on gluten-free fried bread ***
So as to avoid the bread taking up too much oil, toast lightly first. Heat a tablespoon of sunflower oil in a frying pan. Put in the bread, frying it quickly on one side only until crisp. Keep warm on a warm plate while you fry the egg on one or both sides, whichever is preferred. Put the egg on to the fried side of the bread and serve.

Soft-boiled egg ****
For a soft-boiled egg put enough hot water into a small

saucepan that you think will cover the egg and bring to the boil. Take off the heat and lower an egg into the water on a teaspoon. Put back over the heat and boil steadily for 3 minutes for a medium egg and 4 minutes for a large. Serve in an egg cup with fingers ('soldiers') of gluten-free bread, fresh or toasted.

COLD BREAKFASTS

Hard-boiled egg ****
Use the same method as for soft boiled but allow 10 minutes and then plunge the egg into cold water. Let the egg cool for a minute then tap with a spoon to fracture the shell. Peel off the shell and membrane underneath. Wash under the cold tap to remove all traces of shell. To move it about, put into small dish. To eat, cut it up on a plate, season to taste and serve with gluten-free bread or toast and margarine.

Muffins – see chapter 10 for these, both savoury and semi-sweet.

Flying starts (makes 10) *****
These are for people who don't have time to sit down to a breakfast. They are a kind of muesli made into a cookie and have the advantage of being suitable to break into pieces and use as a breakfast cereal. Nutritious and filling.

    3 oz (75g) RG77 gluten-free flour blend
    2 pinches Xanthan gum
    ½ level teaspoon gluten-free baking powder
    1 oz (25g) polyunsaturated soft margarine
    2 heaped teaspoons brown sugar or 1 generous teaspoon
        runny honey
    1 heaped teaspoon low fat milk powder

1 oz (25g) freshly ground mixed nuts – hazelnuts, walnuts,
  almonds, brazils (but not peanuts)
1 medium egg beaten with 3 drops of vanilla flavouring
1 level tablespoon each of sultanas and raisins and
  2 chopped dried apricots
1 small eating apple, peeled, cored and chopped small
  seeds for finishing – sesame, linseeds, sunflower seeds

Method: Preheat oven at Gas 5/190 °C/375 °F. Line a
baking sheet with baking parchment. Put the flour into a
bowl with the Xanthan gum and baking powder. Add the
margarine and rub in with the fingers until the mixture
resembles fine crumbs. Sprinkle in the sugar (or drizzle in
the honey) and the milk powder, add nuts and fruit. Mix by
hand to distribute evenly. Pour in the egg mixture and work
it in with a metal spoon. (Keep going, it will go in completely without any more liquid.) When it has gone into 1
lump, wet your hands and break off pieces about the size of
a large walnut. Shape each one into a sausage and flatten.
Sprinkle seeds over the tops, if using, and bake on the top
shelf for about 20 minutes or until golden. Cool on a wire
rack. When cold individually wrap in food film and store in
an airtight container. Use within a week. 2 or 3 will make a
breakfast.
  Note: Destoned, chopped prunes can also be used in the
dried fruit mixture.

Flying Start cereal (1 serving) *****
Slice thinly then chop 2 or 3 Flying Starts and put into a bowl
with a little fresh fruit of some kind – 2 or 3 strawberries or
blueberries etc. Pour over a little cold milk and serve.

Muesli (serves 1) *****
Peel and core a ripe eating apple. Cut into thin slices and put

into a serving bowl. Sprinkle with the following: 1 level table-spoon of chopped nuts, 1 heaped teaspoon of raisins or sultanas, 1 heaped tablespoon of cold boiled rice and a sprinkle of brown sugar. Stir and pour over a little cold milk. 2 dried apricots, chopped, and a sprinkle of sesame and sunflower seeds can also be used.

SNACKS

Don't just reach for the junkfood as there are alternatives which are much healthier. Soups, filled baps, sandwiches, burgers, scones, milk shakes, vegetable dips, homemade cookies ...

Soups – see chapter 5.
Filled gluten-free baps and sandwiches – see chapter 3
    for the baps and chapter 11 for fillings.
Beefburgers and vegetarian burgers – see chapter 7
Scones – see chapter 3
Milk shakes – see chapter14
Snacks on toast

Cheese on toast ✳✳✳
Cover gluten-free toast with finely grated low fat cheddar cheese. Put under a hot grill to melt and bubble. Serve immediately. Good with soup, cut into fingers.

Cheese and tomatoes on toast ✳✳✳✳
Make cheese on toast but grill only for a minute. Cover with slices of tomato and put back under the grill for another 2 or 3 minutes. Make sure the slices of tomato cover the cheese completely or the edges will burn. Serve immediately.

Mushrooms on toast ****
Fry 2 oz (50g) sliced mushrooms in 2 teaspoons margarine.
Season to taste with salt and freshly ground black pepper.
Serve hot on gluten-free toast and eat immediately.

Pâté on toast ****
Serve any of the pâtés in this book, spread on hot gluten-free
toast. Garnish with a fresh tomato and either a few sprigs of
watercress or 2 or 3 lettuce leaves.

Egg on cheese on toast ***
Make cheese on gluten-free toast and top with a poached egg.
Serve immediately.

NIBBLES

Chapati crisps *****
Make chapatis – (see chapter 3). Break into small pieces.
They can be flavoured with 3 pinches mild curry powder for
variety. Serve on a saucer or in a small bowl.

Cheese straws ***
Use leftover shortcrust pastry (see chapter 3). Roll out on
food film dusted with rice flour. Cut in half. Spread one piece
with a little gluten-free ready- made mustard. Sprinkle with
finely grated Parmesan cheese. Cover with the second piece
of pastry and roll the rolling pin over them to press the two
pieces and the filling together. Place upside down on a
greased baking sheet and peel off the food film. Cut into thin
straws with a sharp knife. Bake in a preheated oven at Gas
7/200 °C/425 °F on the top shelf for about 8 – 10 minutes,
until golden. Leave to cool on the baking sheet. As they cool
down they will become crisp. Serve in a bowl. Store in plastic bag, sealed.

Snax ***

Crisp and crunchy to eat with drinks or for a party. Make crispy noodles (see chapter 3) but before frying, cut into short lengths. Drain on kitchen paper and sprinkle with a little salt. Store in a sealed plastic bag until you are ready to use.

Toasted nuts *****

Put whole almonds into a sponge tin and bake near the top of the oven for 6 minutes at Gas 6/200 °C/400 °F. Put into a small bowl when cold.

Pizza

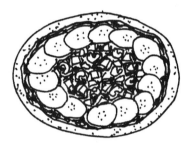

This can be eaten as a snack if it is small or a larger size for a main meal It can be a cheap, healthy food made at home or an expensive high calorie, grossly high fat, junkfood when made commercially. It is basically hot food on a plate you can eat. A variety of topping ingredients can be used – meat, fish, vegetables and herbs with a light finish of cheese. A good pizza with a green side salad and fresh fruit to follow can make a good, healthy main meal. For a snack it can be eaten on its own. It needs to be eaten freshly made and doesn't lend itself to reheating. Pizza is always a cheerful food on account of its colours, to be eaten any time of day – breakfast, elevenses, brunch, lunch, tea, dinner or supper. It will even make an appearance at parties in miniature form or small slices, and at barbequeues. However, it does not make a good packed lunch as it needs to be eaten as soon as it is cooked.

The base
The base – which should be rolled out or pressed out quite thin with the fingers – can be made of uncooked bread dough or scone dough. (Both of these are in chapter 3.) An edge needs to be raised all round to contain the topping. The base is covered in tomato slices, an Italian tomato sauce,or canned chopped, peeled plum tomatoes. On top of this, scattered about or arranged, goes the protein and sliced or chopped vegetables. Finely grated cheese is scattered over the top and the pizza is put into a hot oven to bake quickly. This makes the retaining edge crisp and cooks the filling. The base must be gluten-free, also the Italian sauce – see chapter 8.

Toppings ****
Here is a list of suggestions for the toppings. Use 1 of the protein foods but 3 or 4 of the vegetables and always a light sprinkling of either finely grated Parmesan or low fat, tasty cheddar which helps to keep the topping moist.

Protein: drain a can of sardines in oil, cut into small pieces/ drain and flake drained canned tuna in oil/ trim back bacon of fat, grill or fry and cut the lean into small squares with kitchen scissors / chop pieces of cooked chicken into small pieces/ trim fat off ham (without breadcrumb coating) and cut into small pieces.

Vegetables: all colours of pepper, chopped/ chopped celery, mushrooms, cucumber, cooked green beans/thinly sliced courgettes/finely chopped onion/cooked shredded leeks/ defrosted frozen peas/sliced boiled potato.

Herbs/garnish: 1 clove of garlic put through a crusher/ stoned black olives, halved/basil leaves, torn into small pieces (or pinches of dried).

Pizza with topping

Method: Preheat oven at Gas 7/220 °C/425 °F. Prepare the tomatoes, protein and vegetables of your choice Make the base of your choice – either bread or scone dough. Grease a baking sheet. Put the dough in the centre and roll out with a rolling pin or press out with the fingers. Raise a slight edge all round. Cover the base with tomato. Arrange the protein. Scatter or arrange with the vegetables and herb/garnish. Sprinkle on the cheese and bake on the top shelf for about 15 minutes or less until the edge is golden and the top sizzling. Serve on a warm plate.

Breakfast pizza (serves 1) ****

See chapter 3 for pizza base recipe and this chapter for instructions. A suitable topping for breakfast would be chopped ham (without breadcrumb coating) and mushrooms gently fried in a little sunflower oil, spread over the tomato base and topped with a little finely grated low fat cheddar cheese. This can be topped with a poached or scrambled egg.

Cheese and biscuits ****

See chapter 3 for gluten-free crispbreads and crackers. Serve with cheese of your choice, celery sticks, radishes, tomatoes or gluten-free chutney. If fat is a problem there are low- fat versions of hard cheese in supermarkets. Low-fat cottage cheese is also available.

Vegetable Dips (makes a good healthy starter, snack or party fare) *****

Wonderful bite-sized pieces of fresh vegetables for dipping into an appetizing sauce. (See Chapter 8 for suggestions)

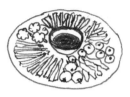

Freshly prepared, they are a good source of vitamins – about as healthy and varied as you can get. Here is a selection of suitable vegetables. Three or four at a time will be sufficient and they will change with the seasons. Keep your selection as colourful as possible. Avoid frozen vegetables as they are not suitable.

Carrot: scrub, peel, trim and cut into small sticks

Radishes: top and tail, cut in half or leave whole

Spring onions: choose small ones, wash and trim so a little of the tender green is left on

Celery: wash and trim, cut into small sticks

Cauliflower: if daisy fresh and crisp, wash and cut into florets

Pepper: use red and yellow for colour, wash and cut out the stem and seeds, cut into strips

Watercress: wash thoroughly and break into sprigs

Courgettes: wash but don't peel, cut into small sticks

Lettuce: wash small heart leaves of crisp lettuce such as Little Gem

Fennel: wash, trim, pull off a layer and cut into small curved sticks

Tomatoes: use small tomatoes, wash and leave whole

See chapter 8 for a selection of gluten free dipping sauces. Mayonnaise type or salad dressings are all suitable. If eating at home serve in a small dish surrounded by the prepared vegetables. For taking to a party or for a picnic, a small screwtop jar is preferable for the sauce dip, and the prepared vegetables in an airtight container.

Probably the best kind of snack, the easiest and the healthiest is a piece of fruit. Some fruits like the banana and clementines come already packaged.

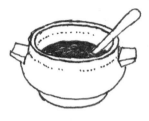

CHAPTER 5

Soups and Starters

Soup has come down to us as a very ancient form of hot food, made in a pot on the edge of an open fire with ingredients that had been foraged for free. Eventually it came to be known as potage. The foraging still goes on but nowadays it takes place in the supermarket and we have to pay.

Soup will warm you up on a cold day and help to fill you up. Some soups are equivalent to a main course and others are merely an appetizer for food to come. It is no surprise then, to find supermarket shelves stocked with all kinds of convenience soup – packet mixes, cartons and tins – just add water, heat or just open and stick in the microwave. They always taste the same as they are made from formulas. They will all have been processed weeks, months or even years before. Most will have a long list of ingredients which can include gluten. It will probably be in the thickener and the stock, flavour enhancers such as MSG (which can be made from wheat), colourings and all kinds of ingredients you would not dream of putting into homemade soup.

Gluten-free soup is very easy to make at home. Colour,

flavour, aroma and texture all play a part in its attraction and all kinds of ingredients can be used. Vegetables, meat, poultry, fish, seasoning, herbs, a gluten-free stock and sometimes a gluten- free thickener are the basics.

The most popular soups have not changed for decades – tomato, mushroom and chicken. As a wide range of ingredients is available all year round there are many other options – asparagus, watercress, celery, peppers etc.

Stock: Soup without stock can be just a tasteless liquid but stock will give it body and bring out the flavour of the ingredients. See chapter 2 for details.

Thickener: Some soups magically thicken themselves as they cook. Others need a little cornflour or potato and a few don't need any thickening as it would give them the wrong texture. None of it is a problem with gluten-free soup if you make it at home.

Variety: While some soups have just one obvious ingredient such as chicken or tomato, others have a variety of ingredients such as minestrone, a mixed vegetable soup. Usually the name of the soup indicates its feature ingredient. Actually, the main ingredient in a soup is water from the tap and this is why soup is not an expensive food.

Equipment: A blender (liquidizer) will reduce cooked soup ingredients to a liquid in seconds, albeit in an earsplitting way. A mouli, by contrast is worked by hand and is quite quiet, The cooked pieces to be processed are pushed through a metal plate with holes into a bowl underneath. I use both a blender and a mouli in my kitchen. Both are messy but the end result is worth it.

What to eat with soup

Croûtons – Cut a slice of gluten-free bread. Cut into fingers and then across to make small cubes. Fry in a little hot oil for a minute then turn with a spatula and fry a little more until

crisp. Take out of the pan with a spatula and put on to kitchen paper to drain. Scatter into soup just as you serve. ***
Oven scones – make these without sugar.
Bread, rolls, farls, savoury muffins, breadsticks – see chapter 3 for recipes.

Tomato Soup (2 servings) ****

½ medium onion, chopped
2 teaspoons sunflower oil
½ medium can chopped peeled plum tomatoes
½ pint (300ml) water
3 pinches sugar (or to taste)
2 teaspoons gluten-free soy sauce or stock of your choice
    salt and freshly ground black pepper to taste
either 5 sprigs of parsley or 5 leaves of basil, finely
    chopped

Method: Gently stir/fry the onion in the oil, using a medium sized pan, for 5 minutes, until soft but not browned. Put the tomatoes, water and cooked onion into the blender and blend. Pour back into the pan and heat through, adding the gluten-free stock. Stir in and season to taste with sugar, salt and freshly ground black pepper. Stir in the basil if using and serve hot. If using parsley, sprinkle a little into each bowl before serving.

Note: If serving for a special meal, omit herbs and drizzle in half a tablespoon of single cream to each bowl to make **cream of tomato soup.** ***

Red pepper and tomato soup (2 servings) ****

½ medium onion, finely chopped
1 tablespoon extra virgin olive oil

1 clove garlic, put through a crusher
1 medium red pepper, deseeded and stalk cut out, chopped
    small
4 peeled medium tomatoes, canned or fresh caster sugar to
    taste
2-3 teaspoons gluten-free soy sauce or stock of your
    choice
½ pint (300ml) water
2 heaped teaspoons finely chopped fresh parsley
salt and freshly ground black pepper to taste

Method: Fry the onion lightly in the oil over a medium heat.
Crush in the garlic and stir. Put in the red pepper, tomatoes,
2 pinches sugar, soy sauce and about 2/3 of the water. Bring
to the boil and lower heat to simmer for about 15 minutes.
Add the rest of the water and pour into the blender. Liquidize
and return to pan. Sprinkle in the parsley. Taste and season
with salt and pepper; adjust sugar and stock to taste.

Watercress soup (2-3 servings)
A quickly made, dark green soup, thickened with potato and
full of goodness.

½ medium onion, finely chopped
1 oz (25g) polyunsaturated soft margarine
¾ pint (425ml) water
1 bunch fresh watercress
1 slightly heaped tablespoon cooked potato, chopped or
    mashed
2–3 teaspoons gluten-free soy sauce or stock of your
    choice salt to taste

Method: Put the watercress into a bowl of cold water. Discard
any yellowing or bruised leaves. Inspect closely for foreign

bodies. Shake and put on to a chopping board. Chop coarsely including the stems. Fry the onion gently in the margarine for 5 minutes but don't let it brown. Put about half the water into the liquidizer goblet with the prepared watercress and mashed potato. Add the cooked onion and blend. Pour into the pan with the rest of the water and the soy sauce. Bring to the boil and lower the heat to simmer for a further 5 minutes. Season to taste with salt. Serve hot in the winter and cold from the fridge in summer.

Pea soup (2 servings) ****
This delightful green soup has a little protein to offer.

½ medium onion, chopped finely
2 teaspoons sunflower oil
just under ½ pint (300ml) water
6 oz (175g) frozen peas
2 teaspoons gluten-free stock or stock of your choice
salt and freshly ground black pepper

Method: Fry the onion in the oil until transparent but do not let it brown. Pour in half the water, put in the peas and stock. Gently bring to the boil.

On a lower heat, simmer for 5 or 6 minutes. Add the remaining water, pour into the liquidizer and blend.. Heat and add seasoning to taste. Serve.

Mushroom soup (2 servings) ****
Quick to make and very tasty.

½ medium onion, chopped finely
2 teaspoons sunflower oil
2 oz (50g) mushrooms, sliced thinly
just under ½ pint (300ml) water

2 heaped teaspoons dried milk powder
2 teaspoons gluten-free soy sauce or stock of your choice
salt and freshly ground black pepper

Method: Gently stir/fry the onion in the oil, using a medium sized pan, for 5 minutes until soft but not browned. Put the raw mushrooms into the blender with the water, milk and stock. Blend and pour into the pan. Bring to the boil then lower heat to simmer for 5 minutes. Taste and season. Serve hot.

Parsley Soup (2-3 servings) *****
If you haven't been eating up your greens, this is the answer as it is extremely good for you. It is thickened by the addition of potato.

1 heaped teaspoon polyunsaturated soft margarine
½ medium onion, sliced
2 oz (50g) fresh parsley, finely chopped
2 teaspoons gluten-free soy sauce or stock of your choice
1 small potato, peeled and thinly sliced
1 pint (600ml) skimmed milk
salt and freshly ground black pepper

Method: Fry the onion gently in the margarine for 5 minutes, with the lid on. Add the potato and parsley and cook/stir for 2 minutes. Put in the milk and soy sauce. Bring almost to the boil then lower heat to simmer for about 25 minutes with the lid on. Take off the heat and allow to cool for a few minutes before pouring into the liquidizer. Blend and return to pan. Taste and season, adding a little water if it has turned out too thick, and more of the stock if required. Can be served hot in winter or cold in summer from the fridge.

Pea and Asparagus Soup (2 servings) ****

¼ medium sized onion, finely chopped
1 tablespoon sunflower oil
2 oz (50g) trimmed, fresh asparagus (about 8 medium
    spears)
1½ oz (40g) frozen peas
½ pint (300ml) water
3 teaspoons gluten-free soy sauce
salt and freshly ground black pepper

Method: Using a small pan, gently fry the onion in the oil for
5 minutes. Chop the asparagus into short lengths and put into
the pan with the peas and about 2/3 of the water. Bring to the
boil then lower heat for about 7-8 minutes, until the vegetables are tender. Add the soy sauce and remaining water. Pour
into the liquidizer and blend. Pour back into the pan and bring
to the boil. Season to taste and serve. For a special occasion
swirl a little single cream into each serving. ***

Vegetable soups – a good way to eat more vegetables.
Homemade mixed vegetable soups are never the same twice
and they are much more likely to be seasonal. This adds variety. (Commercial soups are the same all year round, year in
year out.) As all vegetables are naturally gluten-free they
should play a useful part in a gluten-free diet. Here is a list of
suitable vegetables and herbs etc. from which to choose. The
vegetables starred are those best used in small amounts.
*****

Onion, spring onions
Carrot, swede, turnip, parsnip, celeriac
*Spinach, mushrooms, courgettes
*Cabbage, * greens

Peppers, tomatoes (canned or fresh)
Broad beans, green beans, runner beans
Peas, leeks, lettuce, cucumber
Watercress, cucumber
*Garlic, parsley,
Chives, *sage, mint, basil, marjoram
Mild gluten-free curry powder can also be used, also
    tomato purée

(I have left off the following as they can be rather overpowering in flavour : sprouts, broccoli, beetroot, fennel, sprout tops and cauliflower.) Avoid a taste battle and just use about 5 or 6 different vegetables for a mixed vegetable soup.

Vegetable broth and stock *****

This thin soup is not only comforting when you are ill but has good levels of potassium. Make a large pan of it and use on the day of making. Any left over can be frozen in an ice cube tray and use as required for stock.

2 medium onions, sliced
a selection of vegetables – what you have in the kitchen –
    chopped small to ¾ fill a medium sized pan, about
    1½ lbs (750g). It should include coarsely grated carrots
    and celery
boiling water – about 2 pints (1 litre) or more to cover the
    vegetables
gluten-free soy sauce or stock of your choice
tomato purée (optional)
salt and freshly ground black pepper

Method: Put the onions and other prepared vegetables into a medium sized pan with the water and bring to the boil. Put the lid on slightly to one side to let out the steam and lower the heat to simmer for about 30 – 40 minutes and check every 10 minutes to see if more hot water is required. When the vegetables are disintegrating and all their goodness has gone into the liquid, set a large colander over a bowl and spoon in the contents of the pan. Allow the cooked vegetables to drain for a few minutes then discard, saving the juices in the bowl. Pour into the pan and reheat. Stir in a tablespoon of gluten-free soy sauce or stock of your choice and a heaped teaspoon tomato purée if you wish. Season to taste with salt and pepper. Serve hot. Can be served as a drink in a mug.

Notes: If you want to save time on the simmering, grate all the root vegetables and finely chop/shred the others. Cut 15 minutes from the cooking time.

If you want to make a **mixed vegetable soup**, halve the amounts. Simmer for only 20 minutes and after leaving to cool for 5 minutes, blend or put through a mouli. Return to pan and add 2 teaspoons gluten-free soy sauce or stock of your choice. Season with salt and freshly ground black pepper. To make it more interesting put in a few pinches mixed herbs or gluten-free mild curry powder, tomato purée and/or 2 teaspoons single cream.

Minestrone – 2 generous servings *****
This classic, hearty soup is enough for a main meal if the beans or peas are included.

1 tablespoon extra virgin olive oil
½ medium onion, finely chopped
1 stick celery, chopped
1 small leek, slice thinly
½ medium carrot, coarsely grated
1 clove garlic put through a crusher
½ medium can, chopped, peeled plum tomatoes
½ pint (300ml) water

1 tablespoon gluten-free soy sauce or stock of your choice
2 cabbage leaves, shredded finely, main stalks removed
1½ oz (40g) uncooked, gluten-free spaghetti, broken into
    short lengths
1½ oz (40g) canned, gluten-free haricot beans or frozen peas
1 heaped teaspoon fresh, finely chopped parsley
salt and freshly ground black pepper to taste
grated Parmesan cheese to serve

Method: Heat the oil in a medium saucepan and stir/fry the
onion, celery, leek, carrot and garlic for 5 minutes. Add the
tomatoes, water, stock, cabbage and beans or peas. Bring to
the boil, lower heat and simmer with the lid on for about 10
-12 minutes. Put in the spaghetti, stir and cook for another 10
minutes. Add the parsley, stir and serve hot with a sprinkle of
Parmesan.

Note: If you don't want to use beans or frozen peas, use
kitchen scissors to cut the lean from 2 slices back bacon. Cut
into small squares and lightly fry in a teaspoon of olive oil for
a minute. Use instead of the beans or peas. Other beans to use
are butter beans and red kidney beans. Both can be bought
ready cooked in cans. Check labels before buying/using.

STARTERS

Parma ham and melon (1 serving) ****
This is a stylish looking starter that always appears enviable.
It is very quick to make.

¼ medium sized, ripe melon
2 – 3 thin slices Parma ham

Method: Cut away and discard the melon seeds. Cut the flesh
away from the skin and slice into long slices, the length of the

melon. Lay on a plate and cover with the Parma ham. Serve with a small knife and fork.

Note: If the melon turns out to be not sweet enough, sprinkle with a few pinches of caster sugar. If melons are out of season, use ripe kiwi fruit. Peel off the brown skin and cut into thin slices.

Papaya and prawns (1 serving) ****

    1 ripe papaya
    1 heaped tablespoon defrosted or fresh prawns (small)
    1 tablespoon light gluten-free mayonnaise – see chapter 8

Cut a ripe papaya in half, lengthways. Use a teaspoon to scoop out and discard the seeds, leaving a cavity. Put the prawns into a small basin with the mayonnaise. Turn over with a spoon to coat then fill the cavity in the papaya, heaping the prawns up. Use a sprig of watercress or parsley to serve.

Avocado and orange with sesame dressing – (1 serving) *****

The dressing will stop the avocado from discolouring so have it ready before you start peeling. This looks very good served on white tea plates. Simple, stunning and gluten-free.

    1 ripe avocado
    1 sweet, juicy orange
    1 tablespoon sesame oil dressing – see chapter 8
    freshly ground black pepper

Method: Halve then peel the avocado and remove the stone. Cut out the flesh in small scoops with a teaspoon and pile on to 2 teaplates. Peel the orange with a sharp serrated knife, cutting away the peel and pith. Cut the segments away from the membranes. Arrange on top of the avocado. Wring out the orange membranes over a small bowl before discarding as there will be juice still left in them. Add the sesame oil dressing and mix. Drizzle over the avocado and orange. Finish with a grind of black pepper. Serve with a gluten-free roll to mop up the juices.

Melon *****
Serve a wedge of melon. Cut a segment out of a ripe fruit, cut away the seeds but leave the outer skin on. With a sharp knife loosen the flesh on each side. Cut 3 lines down through the flesh lengthways and then lines across to make cubes. Alternatively, remove the cubes and put into a glass dish with a teaspoon. Little balls can be made with a melon baller but this method tends to be wasteful. There are usually several kinds of melon at the supermarket – Cantaloupe, Charentais etc. The sweetest and ripest ones will be the heaviest fruit. They will also smell of melon.

Fruit plate *****
A plate with a display of fresh fruit always looks colourful and attractive. Use ripe, sweet fruit. Melon, papaya, orange, halved seedless grapes, destoned cherries, sliced destoned ripe plums, and fresh pineapple can all be used. Only use a small helping of each one and about 4 is plenty. Arrange on a white plate. To finish, squeeze over a passion fruit or make some raspberry sauce – see chapter 8.

Pâtés ****
Who knows what goes into the average commercial pate? The prepacked kind make interesting reading but the ones sold loose off the deli counter don't have this advantage. Wheat flour, rusk, MSG which could be made from wheat starch, and who knows what else. Make your own pâté at home and

avoid the worry. Pâtés can be made from nuts as well as meat and poultry. Herbs, mushrooms tomato purée and spices can be added for extra flavour. A small food processor is essential to make them.

Walnut pâté *****

    1 spring onion, trimmed and finely chopped
    3 teaspoons sunflower oil
    1 teaspoon gram flour
    4 tablespoons water
    2 heaped tablespoons ground walnuts
    1 heaped teaspoon gram flour
    4 tablespoons water
    3 pinches dried thyme or ¼ teaspoon finely chopped fresh
    1 level teaspoon tomato purée
    few drops fresh lemon juice
    freshly ground black pepper to taste

Method: Use a small frying pan to stir/fry the onion in the oil for half a minute. Add the gram flour and mix well to absorb the oil. Continue to stir/fry over a gentle heat. Add the water and cook while you stir for 3 minutes, until you have a stiff paste. Take off the heat and stir in the nuts, thyme, tomato puree and lemon juice. If it feels too stiff add a little more water. Season to taste and turn into a small dish to grow cold. Cover and store in the fridge. Eat within 3 or 4 days. Serve with gluten-free toast or fresh baked gluten-free rolls. See chapter 3.

Chicken liver pâté (2 or 3 servings) *****

    8 oz (225g) chicken livers, chopped finely
    1 shallot or ¼ of a small onion

1 tablespoon extra virgin olive oil
½ clove garlic put through a garlic press
1 pinch dried mixed herbs or ½ teaspoon fresh chopped
freshly ground black pepper
2 heaped teaspoons low fat dried milk powder dissolved in
    1 tablespoon water
1 teaspoon sherry
2 teaspoons gluten-free soy sauce

Method: Wash the chicken livers and pick them over, discarding any stringy or yellow parts. Chop. Fry the onion in the oil for about 4 minutes while stirring. Crush in the garlic then put in the liver, herbs and seasoning to taste. Stir/fry using a wooden spoon to break up the livers as they cook. After about 5 minutes they should be crumbly and have changed colour. Allow to cool a little then put into a blender with the milk, sherry and soy sauce. Blend to a thick paste. If it turns out too thin, put back into the pan and heat while you stir to reduce. Spoon into a dish. Cover and store in the fridge. Eat within 3 days. Serve with gluten-free toast.

Prawn cocktail *(*1 serving) ****
A very pretty starter, mostly pink and green.

3 or 4 lettuce leaves, torn into small pieces
1 fresh tomato
1 heaped tablespoon fresh or defrosted small prawns
1 generous tablespoon gluten-free pink mayonnaise (made
    with gluten-free light mayonnaise – see chapter 8)
5 thin slices cucumber

Method: Line a glass dessert dish with the lettuce to make a bed. Cut the tomato into wedges and place them around the edge of the lettuce. Coat the prawns with the mayonnaise and

pile in the centre. Decorate with the cucumber, round the
edge, and garnish with the parsley sprig. Serve with gluten-
free bread and butter or a freshly baked gluten-free roll.

Other starters to consider are fresh fruit juices and fruit
kebabs – see fruit in chapter 9.

Stuffed mushrooms (serves 1 for a main meal or 2 as a snack
or starter) ***

    2 large cup-shaped mushrooms
    1 tablespoon sunflower oil
    ¼ medium onion, chopped finely
    ½ clove garlic put through a crusher
    1 heaped tablespoon gluten-free breadcrumbs (see note
        below)
    2 slices back bacon, lean only, cut into small squares
    1 tablespoon chopped fresh parsley
    1 tablespoon finely grated Parmesan cheese or
        finely grated, tasty low-fat cheddar cheese
    salt and freshly ground black pepper
    parsley sprigs for garnish (optional)

Method: Wash the mushrooms and pull out the stalks. Finely
chop stalks. Grease a shallow ovenproof dish. Fry the onion
gently in the oil for 3 minutes. Crush in the garlic, add the
bacon, mushroom stalks and breadcrumbs. Stir/fry gently for
about 4 minutes. Stir in the parsley and cheese. Season to
taste. Put the mushroom caps into the dish, hollow side up.
Fill with the stuffing mixture. Cover loosely with foil or
baking parchment and cook in a preheated oven at Gas 5/190°
C/375° F above centre shelf for about 25 minutes. Serve hot,
garnished with parsley. For a main meal serve with vegetables. For a starter serve on their own.

Note. Make your own gluten-free breadcrumbs with an electric coffee grinder. Blitz small pieces of gluten-free bread.

Vegetable dips – see chapter 4

Make light lunches out of the soups with a sandwich and a piece of fruit.

The starters also will make a light lunch.

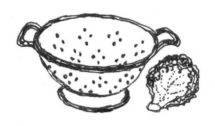

CHAPTER 6

Vegetables

All plain fresh and frozen vegetables are gluten-free. They form an important part of the diet as they provide many of the essential vitamins, minerals and trace elements for a healthy lifestyle. The average person doesn't seem to have the faintest idea of the importance of vegetables as they prefer to rely on junkfood. The basic list of what is available offers an amazing variety for colour, appearance, taste and nutritional value. They all start out as gluten-free although processing, and cooking can allow gluten to get a foothold. Some vegetables can be eaten raw, others can be cooked as well as eaten raw. Vegetables are generous with fibre, carbohydrate, vitamins, minerals and a little protein, but no fat to speak of. They taste nice, look nice, smell nice, are sold in every supermarket and are cheap. Why are they so unpopular?

Here is a basic list of vegetables that can be eaten raw or cooked:

onions, spring onions, fennel
carrot, swede, turnip, parsnip
celery, celeriac
mushrooms, courgettes, cauliflower
peppers, tomatoes,
runner, string or green beans
lettuce, watercress, beetroot, cucumber

The following need to be cooked:

greens – cabbage, spring greens, sprout tops, kale, spinach,
   broccoli
leeks, peas, potatoes, asparagus, garlic, beansprouts
beans – runner, green, string, broad

Some foods, such as salad leaves, are only eaten raw. The most important vegetables are the ***greens.*** Everyone should have at least one portion of one of these, **every day**. (For more information on the nutritional value of vegetables, see chapter 13.)

There are many options for the supply of vegetables to your kitchen. Fresh, canned, frozen, from the garden, the market, the supermarket, delivered organic boxes etc. They may need preparation, be ready-prepared, or require defrosting. However they enter your home they may need to be prepared, boiled, stir-fried, steamed, fried, baked (roasted), made into soup and drinks or left raw. They may also need to be scrubbed, or peeled, sliced, grated, mashed and chopped. It all depends on the vegetable and it really is more interesting than just opening a tin of baked beans.

Shopping for vegetables
Buy the best you can afford, opt for the freshest, brightest and the ones that look as if they have some life in them. Avoid

over-date, wilting, sweaty or dry looking vegetables as they should go for compost, not into your fridge or vegetable basket. When you are buying greens they should squeak when you squeeze them, even inside a plastic bag. Colours should be bright, not fading or yellowy. Don't buy vegetables that are drooping or are not firm and try not to buy too far in advance. *The fresher they are the better.*

Storage
There is no need to put absolutely everything into the fridge, especially the vegetables that just need to be kept in the dry like onions. Potatoes need to be kept in the dark to stop them turning green or sprouting. A fridge is not a cool, dry store. It is rather a damp, very cold store. Avoid storing vegetables for too long – it is better to buy little and often.

Healthy?
Ready-to-cook vegetables from supermarkets, in plastic bags, sliced and grated might be convenient but they are not necessarily good for your health if they are days old, having had a bath in chlorinated water. As soon as a vegetable is processed like this it begins to lose its vitamin value.

Availability
Out of season, designer vegetables are bound to be more expensive than those in season, especially if they have had to travel from overseas. Sprouts in June and strawberries at Christmas? Local produce, if you can buy it, is bound to be good value as it hasn't had far to travel. Use sell-by dates on packaging to help you decide how fresh produce really is. Farm shops and country markets are worth considering, also delivery to your door of vegetable boxes, especially organic ones.

Preparation

Always wash/scrub vegetables with care, removing any parts you don't want to cook. Pick over leafy vegetables looking for foreign bodies. Coarse leaves cook more easily if the coarsest outer leaves stems are torn away and discarded. Thin leaves such as spinach and watercress need a good swim in a sinkful of water before cooking. Onions, which should feel hard, need the thin papery outside skin removed and the top and bottom cut off. Spring onions need to be trimmed top and bottom. Root vegetables need to be scraped or peeled unless young, trim off tops and bottoms; shell peas, pod broad beans, take the strings off runner beans and slice through diagonally into short pieces; top and tail string beans; cut out the stalk from peppers, including the seeds; cut broccoli and cauliflower into florets; wash beansprouts under the tap in a colander; take off the outer leaves of Brussels sprouts, trim the base and cut a cross into it; trim leeks at the bottom and just above the white part, slice in half lengthways, open out the layers under the cold tap to wash out earth; trim celery top and bottom.

COOKING

Steaming *****

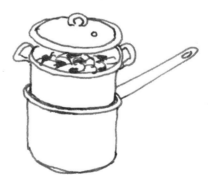

Forget the deep fryer – it isn't a good way to cook. Steaming is a much cleaner and healthier way of cooking and a variety can be cooked at the same time which saves on washing up. You will need a pan half full of boiling water and a steamer which fits into the pan. The bottom of the steamer has holes in it and the water underneath should not be above the holes. The steamer should have a lid to keep the steam in. It works very simply. The water boils in the bottom pan and makes steam. The vegetables are held over it and cook gently in the steam.

The vegetables are not put into the steamer all at the same time as some take longer to cook than others. Root vegetables and cabbage take the longest – about 20 minutes. Carrots sliced quite thinly, turnip, parsnip, swede, and shredded cabbage go in first. After 10 minutes broccoli florets, cauliflower florets and sprouts can be put in, also green beans. After another 7 minutes, slices of courgette, defrosted frozen peas and beansprouts can go in for the last 3 minutes. After a total of 20 minutes all the vegetables are cooked, ready to serve.

If you are making a mixture, 1 root vegetable, cabbage, either broccoli or cauliflower and one 3-minute vegetable will make a good selection. Mixed root vegetables with peas and green beans look very attractive. Slice the root vegetables thinly or they will take too long to steam. Spinach is best just steamed on its own. If you want to boil potatoes at the same time you can put them in the bottom pan. Slice thickly and they too will cook in 20 minutes.

To make bubble and squeak, cook potato slices in the bottom pan and just shredded cabbage in the steamer. (see recipe in chapter 4).

Greens *****
These are so important for a healthy diet. They can all be steamed although kale might take a longer time than 20 minutes. Tear the green off the tough stems and just steam the

green. They can also be boiled. Roll up cabbage leaves and with a large knife slice/cut off shreds. Put these into boiling water to cover and put the lid on. For tender leaves you will need just over 10 minutes, for tougher leaves allow up to 20 minutes. Drain well in a colander. Avoid squelchy greens which can always put people off. Spinach needs only 5 minutes for young leaves and about 10 minutes for tougher leaves. No need to put in more water than a cupful. Drain in a colander and press the back of the spoon into the cooked leaves to get out all the water. If using for ravioli let them grow cold and wring them out in your hand, over the sink. (The way spinach will hang on to water never ceases to amaze. It will never drain left on its own in a colander but always needs persuasion. Press with the back of a spoon if hot.)

Potatoes *****
Never eat potatoes that have gone green. Most of the nutrients in potatoes are stored under the skin so baked potatoes in their jackets (skins) are a good idea and so are new potatoes boiled in their skins. For jacket potatoes good varieties are King Edwards, Desirée, Maris Pipers and Wilgers. They will go soft and fluffy inside and stay crisp-skinned. Prick all over with the point of a knife. They will cook all through if you push a metal skewer right through the middle, lengthways. Give medium sized ones about 50 minutes, large about an hour, in a hot oven on the top shelf.

Jersey Royals are the best new potatoes but wait until they are well into the season before buying as they can be very expensive. Scrub with a nail brush to remove mud and cover with boiling water. Bring back to the boil and cook for about 15 to 25 minutes with the lid on, depending on size.

Mashed potatoes *****
This is best made with old potatoes such as King Edwards.

Cut into thick slices and boil for up to 15 minutes with the lid on. Drain in a colander and put back into the pan. Use a potato masher to purée them, adding a knob of polyunsaturated soft margarine and a little (suitable) milk. Season to taste with salt and freshly ground black pepper with a pinch or two of freshly grated nutmeg. Serve hot or use for cottage pie or fish pie topping and making fishcakes or rissoles.

Three root mash *****
Boil a mixture of potatoes, finely sliced carrots and swede. Cook for 20 minutes and mash as for potatoes. Omit nutmeg. Use as a vegetable or a topping for cottage pie.

1% fat oven chips *****
Forget celebrity chef chips that are deep fried three times, loaded with fat, very high in calories, made in a pan which can catch fire. Some tums cannot cope with such excess. Here is a different kind of chip altogether and it is healthy. At first glance you may think this recipe could not possibly work, but I can assure you it does. After they are cooked they will keep warm for up to 15 minutes in a warm oven.

Use old potatoes, peeled and cut into chips. Allow 1 medium potato per serving. Heat the oven at Gas 8/230° C/450° F. Lightly grease a baking tray with a mere ½ teaspoon of sunflower oil or extra virgin olive oil and put another ½ teaspoon into your palm. Rub your hands together. Turn the chips over, rubbing them through your hands to distribute the oil all over them. Leave them scattered around the edge of the baking tray but not in the centre. Wipe your hands with kitchen paper. Put the chips on the top shelf for 20 – 25 minutes until crisp and golden. Serve immediately if you can.

Stir/stew vegetables *****
This is the easy-peasy way to cook a variety of vegetables and

only have one pan to wash up. It is similar to stir/fry but without such a large amount of fat. The vegetables are quickly and lightly cooked with all their flavours intact and all their juices saved for the gravy. You will need about 4 to 6 different kinds of vegetables for the mix which can be cooked in 10 minutes or less. You will need a large shallow pan with a lid. The vegetables to be used should be prepared before the cooking begins. *Slices should be thin, pieces small and leaves finely shredded.* Start with a spring onion or ¼ of a medium onion, finely chopped.

For one serving put 2 teaspoons sunflower oil into the pan with the onion. Fry gently while you stir for a minute or two then add your prepared vegetables in order of hardness. Root vegetables come first. Stir and put in 2 tablespoons of water. Put the lid on and increase the heat. After 3 or 4 minutes put in the semi-hard vegetables – celery, pepper, peas, greens. Stir again and add more water. Cook for another 3 or 4 minutes and put in the soft vegetables – courgettes, mushrooms, cucumber and bean sprouts. Lower the heat and cook for a mere 2 minutes. When they have cooked, check there is enough liquid in the pan to make the gravy. Stir in 2 teaspoons of gluten-free soy sauce or stock of your choice. This will make the gravy. Serve as soon as you can. Either serve with boiled rice or use thin slices of potato as part of the mix (For the protein part of the meal use any kind of plain baked or poached fish, plain roasted or grilled meat or poultry.)

Note: Whatever your selection of prepared vegetables there should be enough for 1 generous serving per person. Here are some good combinations:

- ¼ medium onion, ¼ medium carrot ½ stick celery, 1 medium mushroom, 1 heaped tablespoon frozen peas (defrosted), 2 broccoli florets

- ¼ medium onion, 2 small potatoes, 1 small leek (put in first), ¼ of a red pepper, 1 medium tomato, juice of ¼ of a lemon – good with chicken
- ¼ medium onion, ½ medium courgette, ¼ pepper, 2 medium tomatoes, 1 medium potato, handful spinach leaves, ½ clove garlic crushed in, 3 sprigs parsley chopped finely – good with fish
- For a Chinese meal – 2 spring onions, ½ stick celery, 5 lettuce leaves (or watercress sprigs), ¼ red pepper, ¼ medium courgette, handful of beansprouts – see chapter 8 for sweet and sour red sauce

Note: Whatever combination of vegetables you use try to get at least one colourful one into it. You will still need to fry onion in oil and add gluten- free stock. For more portions increase the oil, vegetables and gluten-free stock.

Stir/stew is not the same as stir/fry which has much more oil.

SALADS

Salad is not just a side dish for summer. It can go on right through the autumn winter and spring. Salad is not just a couple of lettuce leaves, a tomato and a few slices of cucumber with a blob of commercial dressing. This is an apology for salad and you don't need lettuce for every salad. The real thing is variable, nourishing, easy to prepare and can deliver inspiration. Chapter 8 will give you a range of dressings to use. Here is a list of possibilities for ingredients – it may surprise you.

Leaves – cos lettuce, little gem, round lettuce, (and other varieties but not iceberg) torn; sprigs of watercress, cress, nasturtium, tender spinach, beetroot leaves, rocket, lamb's lettuce, parsley, chives. coriander, red and white cabbage shredded finely.

Roots and stalks – carrots, swede, celeriac, turnip, raw beetroot, (all grated) sliced radishes, chopped spring onion, chopped cauliflower (raw), finely chopped onion, finely sliced green celery, fennel made into matchsticks.

Cooked vegetables: (use when cold)
beetroot, green beans, peas, leeks, potatoes

Fruit and additions:
Wedges of vine tomatoes, thinly sliced courgette, cucumber and peppers, peeled and sliced avocado, garlic

Halved seedless grapes, thinly sliced or chopped eating apples, chopped segments of orange, sultanas, raisins

Chopped walnuts, cashews and almonds, crispy fried bacon and croutons, cold boiled rice.

Putting a mixed salad together
1 leaf, 1 root, 1 stalk, 1 fruit from the lists above *****

Have ready your jar of dressing. Put your choice of pre-pared salad vegetables from the list above, into a bowl. Turn them over gently with your hand, or salad servers. Spoon over the (shaken) dressing of your choice (2 teaspoons per portion) and turn over to coat each vegetable. Serve shortly after making.

Note: Add at least another 2 leafy and root vegetables if you wish.

- A contrast in texture and colour is always more interesting than all the same colour.
- Cooked vegetables are best sprinkled with a little finely chopped onion and an oil based dressing.
- Contrast the colours so salad looks vibrant – contrast light with dark, orange with green and red with yellow.
- put 1 strong flavour with 3 or 4 more subtle ones.

Green salad *****
Cut a clove of garlic in half and rub the cut part all round a
bowl with a pinch of salt and a teaspoon of vinaigrette dressing. Put in mixed lettuce leaves, torn, a few slices of
cucumber, sprigs of watercress and a sprinkle of finely
chopped onion or snipped chives. Add a little more dressing.
Turn over to coat and serve right away.

Purple salad *****
Red cabbage, shredded finely, grated fresh or raw beetroot,
fresh raw grated carrot, finely chopped red onion, tomato cut
into wedges. 2 teaspoons vinaigrette dressing per portion.
Serve up to an hour after it is made.

Coleslaw ****
Finely shredded, crisp cabbage, grated carrot and apple, a few
sultanas. Dress with gluten-free light mayonnaise (see chapter 8).

Potato salad ****
Allow about ½ a medium boiled potato per person. Slice and
chop cold, boiled potatoes and put into a bowl. Add snipped
chives or finely chopped onion to gluten-free light mayonnaise, allowing 1 tablespoon per portion. Mix it into the
potato, turning it over with a spoon to coat. This salad will
wait quite happily in the fridge for about 2 hours, so can be
made in advance.
    See also chapter 8 for more vegetable recipes – soups and
starters.

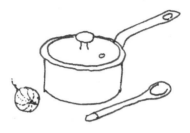

CHAPTER 7

Main Meals

Although grazing on snacks all day and evening seems to be the general direction of Western eating habits, having a main meal each day seems to prevail. The gluten arrives in many disguises, as thickener in stock cubes, gravy mixes, sauces, pastry on top of pies, in dumplings for stews/casseroles, batter for fish, breadcrumb coatings on meat and fish, in sausages with rusk, stuffings, dinner rolls, pasta etc.

The good news is that all plain, fresh and frozen meat, poultry, fish and eggs are gluten-free. (By plain I mean without stuffing or breadcrumb coatings, sauces etc.) There are solutions to all the problems above and they are all simple.

Plain meat and fish can be roasted/baked in the oven, grilled, casseroled/stewed or fried. Eggs are a versatile food that can be boiled, fried, scrambled, poached and pancaked. These are all high protein foods. Cheese and nuts have good levels of protein but also high levels of fat too, so need to be used in small amounts. For more information see chapter 13.

Plain roasted meat * to *****
There are two ways of roasting meat – the high fat way and
the low fat way. The latter is preferable for health. The high
fat way uses lard for a sea of fat with drowning potatoes and
parsnips. There is a better way.
First, choose your joint carefully, as lean as possible. It
should be at room temperature, not cold from the fridge. Put
into a roasting tin and spoon over a tablespoon sunflower oil.
Avoid cooking the potatoes and parsnips in the same tin.
Work out how long the joint will take to roast from the guide
that follows. When the meat is cooked, take it out of the oven,
put on to a warm plate or metal carving dish, turn out the oven
and put the meat back in for a few minutes. See chapter 8 for
how make the gravy with the juices in the roasting tin.

Beef – topside, roast in a preheated oven at Gas 7/225ºC/
425°F, above centre shelf for 15 minutes then turn the
heat down to Gas 5/190°C/375° F for the remainder of
the cooking time. For a rare joint allow 15 minutes per
1lb (450g) plus an extra 15 or 20 minutes. For a
medium joint allow 20 minutes to the 1lb (450g) and 20
minutes extra. See chapter 3 for Yorkshire pudding to
serve with roast beef.

Lamb is best roasted on a metal grid standing in a roasting
tin. Preheat oven at Gas 4/180° C/350°F. Allow 20
minutes per 1lb (450g) and 20 minutes over. Roast
above centre shelf.

Pork needs long cooking over a high heat. It must be
properly cooked right through. Allow 20 minutes to the
1lb (450g) and 25 minutes over at Gas 7/220°C/425°F,
above centre shelf.

Chicken – a 3lb (1.4 kg) oven-ready chicken will take an
hour to roast. Wash out the chicken. Cut lemon into
quarters and fill the cavity.

(Do not fill with stuffing.) Preheat oven at Gas 6/200°C/ 400°F. Grease a roasting tin with sunflower oil. Place the chicken in it, leaning on one side. Roast on a shelf above centre for 20 minutes then turn the chicken on to its other side for another 20 minutes. For the last 20 minutes, turn the chicken upright. A few minutes before the end of the cooking time, prick the bird all over with a fork and let the fat run out.

Mince
The cheapest kind of beef is mince. Only buy 5% fat mince (*****)or the cooked food will be too fatty. Avoid cheap mixtures such as burgers – you just don't know what is in them.

Sausages – Legally, sausages can contain all kinds of things – a little meat, a lot of fat, additives, colourings, flavourings and even bone slurry. A good deal of salt, enhancers and preservatives can help to make sausages the ultimate junk food.

If you make your own at home this culinary minefield will be avoided. This recipe will give you peace of mind and really moreish sausages.

Beef sausages (makes 5-6) ****

1 eating apple, peeled and cored
4 oz (100g) 5% fat, minced beef
1 slice gluten-free bread, made into crumbs
1 small pinch each dried thyme and sage, or 2 pinches each
    of freshly chopped
1 pinch allspice
2 grinds black pepper
¼ teaspoon made gluten-free mustard
2 teaspoons gluten-free soy sauce
½ level teaspoon tomato purée

cornflour (maize) for coating
sunflower oil for shallow frying

Method: Grate the apple finely into a bowl. Add the meat, breadcrumbs, herbs, spice, mustard, soy sauce and tomato puree. Mix everything together with a fork. Flour your hands with cornflour and shape into 5 or 6 sausages. Put a little cornflour on to a plate. Roll the sausages in it to coat all over. Put a tablespoon oil into a frying pan over a medium heat. Put in all the sausages and cook, turning every 2 minutes. When crispy brown and cooked right through (after about 8 minutes), drain on a double thickness of kitchen paper. Serve hot with vegetables or cold with salads.

Pork sausages (makes 5 or 6) ****
Make as for beef sausages but use a pork chop, trimmed of all fat instead of the beef. Change the herbs to just sage and add 1 heaped tablespoon finely chopped onion. Omit the mustard.

Both these sausages make a good sandwich filling – hot or cold with a gluten-free table sauce or gluten-free chutney.

Burgers (makes 2 large or 4 small) ****

6 oz (175g) 5% fat, minced beef
1 slice gluten-free bread made into crumbs
½ medium onion, finely chopped
1 medium egg, whisked in a cup with a fork
freshly ground black pepper
small pinch mixed dried herbs
2 teaspoons gluten-free soy sauce
cornflour for coating
1 tablespoon sunflower oil for frying
gluten-free baps, lettuce and fresh tomato for finishing

Method: Put the first seven ingredients into a bowl and mix well with a fork. Put a little cornflour on to a plate and shape the mixture by hand into flat cakes. Coat, pressing first one side and then the other into the cornflour. Put the oil into a frying pan, over a medium heat. Fry gently on each side for 4 minutes. Drain on kitchen paper to remove excess fat. Serve inside split gluten-free baps with a layer of sliced tomato and a layer of lettuce leaves.

Note: See chapter 3 for baps.

Vegetarian burgers (makes 2) ****
A useful recipe for people who don't like or want to eat meat.

white of 4 spring onions, chopped finely
1 oz (25g) gluten-free breadcrumbs or 1 heaped tablespoon mashed potato
3 teaspoons gluten-free soy sauce
1 heaped teaspoon tomato purée
1 egg, beaten
2 medium tomatoes, finely chopped
3 oz (75g) ground nuts (almonds, hazelnuts, walnuts, brazil nuts)
1 teaspoon fresh mixed herbs, finely chopped (or ½ teaspoon dried)
freshly ground black pepper to taste
rice flour
sunflower oil for frying

Method: Use a fork to mix the first nine ingredients in a bowl. Divide the mixture into four. Flour your hands with rice flour and shape them into cakes. Dust all over with more rice flour and shallow-fry in a little oil for 3 minutes on each side. Serve on a warm plate with broccoli, peas, carrots, cabbage and gravy – see chapter 8.

Pasties (makes 2 large or 4 small) ***
The filling is precooked to save overbaking the pastry. See
chapter 3 for shortcrust pastry.

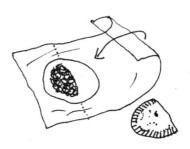

2 teaspoons sunflower oil
1 medium onion, sliced thinly
2 medium potatoes, peeled and cut into thick slices
4 heaped tablespoons 5% fat, minced beef
2 teaspoons gluten-free soy sauce
salt and freshly ground black pepper
rice flour

Method: Preheat oven at Gas 6/200°C/400°F. Boil the potato
slices for 15 minutes then drain and put to one side. Rinse out
the pan and dry with kitchen paper. Lightly fry the onion in
the oil while you stir for 2 minutes. Add the minced beef and
turn over while you cook for 5 minutes. When it has turned
from red to greyish pink add the soy sauce and add salt and
pepper to taste. Put in the potato slices and cut them with a
knife to make smaller pieces. Mix. Put to one side while you
make the shortcrust pastry from chapter 3. Divide the pastry
into the number of pieces you want. Roll each piece out, one
at a time, to one side, of a piece of food film, dusted with rice
flour. Use the filling to make a mound on the left side of the
pastry, leaving space around the edge. Brush the edge with
water. Lift the food film up gently on the right hand side and

fold it up and over the pasty so it encloses the filling and matches the edges. Press all round the edge with your fingers to seal. Crimp between forefinger and thumb or press with the tines of a fork. Cut a slit in the top to let out the steam. Leaving the pasty on the food film, slide it off and on to a greased baking sheet. Make the remaining one (or three) pasties in the same way. (Brush with egg/ water if you want a shiny, golden finish.) Bake on the top shelf for about 20 minutes. Serve hot with vegetables and gravy, or cold with salad. If eating cold, leave to cool on the baking sheet.

Note: Don't overbake or the pastry will be too dry. It should be pale unless you have used the egg glaze. If you don't have the time to make the pasties in the above way just cut two rounds or squares for each one, heap the filling in the middle, brush with water all round and put the second piece of pastry on top. Press all round the edge to seal etc. Cut a slit in the middle and bake. Easy.

Bolognese sauce (2-3 servings) for pasta (see chapter 3) ****
There are many recipes for Bolognese sauce and many variations, including rather rich ones. Few are gluten-free as the traditional thickening is wheat flour. Here's a version that is not too rich and definitely gluten-free. Double the recipe and serve to all the family. Freezes well if you make too much.

1 tablespoon extra virgin olive oil
½ medium onion, finely chopped
lean from 1 slice of back bacon, cut into small squares
1 clove garlic, put through a garlic crusher
1 small carrot, finely grated, or ½ a small courgette finely grated
½ stick celery, chopped small
6 oz(150g) 15% fat, minced beef
1 level teaspoon cornflour (maize)

⅓ pint (400ml) water
½ medium can chopped, peeled plum tomatoes
1 tablespoon gluten-free soy sauce or stock of your choice
1 tablespoon tomato puree
salt and freshly ground black pepper
about 10 fresh basil leaves, chopped, or 1 level teaspoon
    dried
freshly grated nutmeg

Method: Put the oil into a saucepan with the onion, bacon and garlic. Fry/stir gently for 5 minutes. Add the beef and cook until it has turned brown. Stir in the tomatoes. Mix the cornflour with 2 tablespoons cold water, in a cup, and add to the pan. Stir/cook for 2 minutes. Pour in the water and add the tomato purée.

Season with salt and pepper to taste and stir in the basil and 3 pinches nutmeg. Serve hot on gluten-free pasta (see chapter 3) sprinkled with Parmesan cheese, with a green side salad or hot spinach or broccoli, for a satisfying and nutritious main course.

Cottage pie (2 servings)
A healthy gluten-free version of an old favourite.

1 tablespoon sunflower oil
about 5 oz (150g) 5% fat minced beef
1 medium mushroom, chopped
½ level teaspoon finely chopped, fresh, mixed herbs, or 3
    pinches dried
2 slightly heaped teaspoons cornflour
cold water
3 teaspoons gluten-free soy sauce or stock of your choice
2 portions mashed potato
salt and freshly ground black pepper

Method: Preheat oven at Gas 4/180° C/350 °F. Fry the onion in the oil over a medium heat while you stir for about 4 minutes. Add the mince and stir/fry for 5 minutes. Put in the mushroom and herbs. Put the cornflour into a cup with a tablespoon of water. Stir and when smooth put in another 3 tablespoons water and the soy sauce. Stir into the meat mixture and bring to the boil. Lower heat and continue to cook until it has thickened – another 2 or 3 minutes. If you feel it is too thick, add a little more water and stir in. Season to taste then turn into an ovenproof pie dish. Cover with mashed potato, forking it up to make a texture.

Make a hole through the potato to the meat filling, in the centre. Bake for 25 minutes, above centre shelf. The base will be bubbling hot and the potato crisp and golden. Serve with steamed vegetables.

Beef casserole (2 servings) ****
A low fat, gluten-free version of a traditional winter main meal.

1 medium onion, sliced thinly
1 tablespoon sunflower oil
rice flour
about 8 oz (225g) rump steak, trimmed of all fat
about 7 fluid oz (200ml) boiling water
2 medium carrots, trimmed and cut into thick slices
2 medium mushrooms, sliced
3 teaspoons gluten-free soy sauce
1 clove garlic, peeled and put through a garlic crusher
2 heaped tablespoon defrosted frozen peas
salt and freshly ground black pepper

Method: Preheat the oven at Gas 6/200° C/400 °F. Put the onions and oil into a flameproof casserole and stir over a medium heat for abut 4 minutes. Cut the meat into cubes with a sharp knife. Sprinkle with rice flour and turn over to coat completely. Add to the casserole and continue to stir/fry while you turn the meat over. When it has turned from red to a greyish pink, pour in the water. Add the carrots, mushrooms and soy sauce. Increase the heat and add the garlic. Stir in and bring to the boil. Put the lid on the casserole and transfer to the middle shelf of the oven for an hour. Return to the hob. Mix half a level tablespoon rice flour with 2 tablespoons cold water in a cup. When smooth, add two tablespoons of the liquid from the casserole. Stir and pour back into the casserole. Stir with a wooden spoon and bring back to the boil. Turn out the heat when the gravy thickens. Add the peas and season to taste. Serve hot with one of the following: jacket, boiled or mashed potatoes, boiled rice or gluten-free baps or rolls. Steamed cabbage, sprouts, spring greens, spinach or curly kale also make an excellent accompaniment – just one of them will do.

Note: This casserole can be made in advance to be warmed up the following day.

Liver and bacon (serves 1) ****

3 oz (75g) lambs' liver
1 slice unsmoked back bacon
¼ of an onion, sliced thinly
1 tablespoon rice flour
sunflower oil

Method: Pick over the liver and cut out any pipes or strings. Cut into slices and put into a plastic bag with the rice flour. Hold the bag closed and shake to coat the liver. Cut the fat off the bacon. Put a tablespoon of oil into a frying pan and put over a medium heat. Gently fry the onion for about 5 minutes. Put in the liver and the bacon. Fry for 2 minutes and then turn over for another 2 minutes. Put on to a warmed plate while you make the gravy in the pan – see chapter 8. Serve with mashed potato or boiled rice, greens and carrots.

Chicken with herbs and lemon – (1 serving)
A quick no-fuss main meal.

> 2 spring onions, trimmed and chopped small including most of the green
> 2 teaspoons extra virgin olive oil
> 1 small chicken breast, skinned and cut into small pieces
> 2 teaspoons gluten-free soy sauce or stock of your choice
> 1 teaspoon finely chopped fresh mixed herbs – parsley, rosemary and thyme
> finely grated rind of ¼ of a lemon
> hot water
> 2 level teaspoons cornflour mixed into 2 tablespoons cold water
> salt and freshly ground black pepper to taste

Method: Fry the onion in the oil for 2 minutes in a small pan. Add the chicken and stir/fry for 5 minutes or until the chicken is cooked. Put in the soy sauce, lemon rind and about 3 tablespoons hot water. Stir and add the cornflour. Heat while you stir until it thickens. Season to taste. Serve hot with steamed vegetables and boiled potatoes or rice.

Savoury rice (2 servings) ****
This is a useful dish, versatile, colourful and tasty.
It is very easy to make. For the protein use prawns, cooked bacon, ham or chicken cut into small pieces.

> ½ medium onion, finely chopped
> 1 tablespoon sunflower oil or extra virgin olive oil
> 1 medium mushroom, chopped

¼ of a red pepper, deseeded and chopped small
2 heaped tablespoons frozen peas. defrosted
½ stick of celery, chopped small
water
1 teaspoon gluten-free soy sauce
4 oz (100g) protein (see above)
juice of ½ a lemon
2 portions boiled rice
salt and pepper to taste

Method: Use a medium saucepan to lightly fry the onion in
the oil until transparent but not browned. Add the mushroom,
red pepper, peas and celery. Spoon in 2 tablespoons water and
soy sauce. Stir/fry for 5 minutes. Stir in the protein of your
choice, lemon juice and cooked rice. Stir/fry for another 3 or
4 minutes to heat through the protein and season to taste.
Serve hot with either a green side salad or hot broccoli or
spinach.

   Note: Other vegetables to add are 2 green beans, chopped,
a few cooked broad beans, chopped, 1 spear of asparagus,
chopped. For a little contrast add 1 tablespoon raisins with the
mushroom.

FISH

Baked fish (2 servings) *****
The easy, quick way to cook fish, without making the kitchen
reek, is to bake it in a covered dish, in the oven. While it
bakes, steam your vegetables and make a suitable sauce – see
chapter 8.

   soft margarine
2 portions filleted cod, haddock, plaice or salmon
finely grated rind and juice of ½ a lemon

salt and freshly ground black pepper
few sprigs of watercress or parsley for garnish

Method: Preheat the oven at Gas 4/180° C/350° F. Grease a small casserole with soft margarine. Wash the fish under the cold tap and place in the dish. Squeeze over the lemon juice and sprinkle with the rind. Season to taste and put a small knob of margarine on top of both fillets. Put the lid on and bake above centre shelf for 15-20 minutes. Test with a skewer to see if it is done. Serve hot with a gluten-free sauce and steamed vegetables such as spinach, carrots, and broccoli.

Note: For salmon, you can use 2 tablespoons white wine instead of the lemon juice and rind. See chapter 8 for sauces.

Fish casserole with leeks *(2 servings)* *****

3 teaspoons sunflower oil
½ a yellow or red pepper, deseeded and cut into strips
1 medium leek, trimmed and cut into short lengths
½ medium tin chopped, peeled plum tomatoes
about 8 oz (225g) skinned, cod or haddock fillets
juice of ½ a lemon
freshly ground black pepper
1 heaped tablespoon finely chopped fresh parsley

Method: Preheat oven at Gas 4/180° C/350 °F. Heat the oil in a flameproof casserole and put in the leeks and strips of pepper. Stir/cook gently for about 4 minutes. Add the tomatoes and bring to the boil. Stir and lower heat to simmer for another 8-10 minutes. Season with 2 grinds of pepper. Place the fish on top and squeeze over the lemon juice. Sprinkle with the parsley and put on the lid. Transfer to oven, centre shelf. Depending on how thick the fillets are, bake for 15–20 minutes. Serve immediately the fish is cooked, on warm plates. Rice or boiled potato (slices) go well with this colourful dish.

Fish pie (2 servings) ****
This is a dish that can be made ahead and reheated when required. A mixture of fresh and canned fish can be used as the fish is put in a sauce and covered with mashed potato. A variety is always more interesting than all one sort. Leftover poached or baked fish, sardines and tuna (canned in oil and drained), and prawns can all be used to equal 2 portions.

> 2 portions boiled potatoes, mashed with a little margarine
>   and a dash of milk
> white sauce (see chapter 8)
> 1 heaped tablespoon finely chopped fresh parsley
> juice of ¼ of a lemon
> 2 portions mixed fish

Method: Preheat the oven at Gas 6/200° C/400° F. Make the white sauce and stir in the parsley and lemon juice. Grease an ovenproof dish. Put in 3 tablespoons of the sauce. Cover with the mixed fish and spoon over more of the sauce. Cover the top with mashed potato, forking it up to make a texture. Bake on a shelf above centre for about 20 – 25 minutes until the top is crisp and golden. Serve hot with at least 2 of these: spinach, peas, grilled tomatoes, green beans or broccoli.

Fish cakes (2 servings) ****
Providing you don't use too much oil for the frying, these are useful for breakfast, lunch or dinner. For fish choose from fresh or frozen cod, haddock, salmon or sardines in oil (drained well), tuna or canned salmon in water. Make the breadcrumbs in a coffee grinder or small food processor.

about 3 oz (75g) cooked or canned fish, mashed with a
    fork
2 portions mashed potato
1 heaped tablespoon finely chopped fresh parsley
freshly ground black pepper
cornflour for coating
sunflower oil for shallow frying
1 egg, beaten with a fork, in a soup plate
2 slices homemade gluten-free bread made into crumbs

Method: Use a fork to combine the fish and mashed potato in
a bowl. Work in the parsley by hand. Shape into 4 flat cakes.
Put a heaped tablespoon of the cornflour on to a plate. Have
the beaten egg ready and put the breadcrumbs on to a plate.
Dip the fishcakes into the cornflour. Coat both sides. Do the
same with the egg and then the crumbs, making sure they are
coated all over.

Heat 2 tablespoons of the oil in a frying pan. Put in the
fishcakes and cook over a medium heat for about 3 or 4 minutes. Use a spatula to turn them over to cook on the other side.
They should be crisp and golden. Drain on kitchen paper and
serve with peas and grilled tomatoes.

Poached fish (serves 2) *****
The fish will cook quickly in the poaching liquid and can be
served with a sauce. Here are 3 different poaching liquids
from which to choose.

1. ¼ pint (150ml) skimmed milk and half a bay leaf.
   Suitable for cod and haddock.
2. ¼ pint (150ml) water, 1 small glass white wine.
3. ½ pint (300ml) water, ½ stick celery finely sliced, 1
   heaped tablespoon coarsely grated carrot, a few sprigs
   of parsley and a dash of white wine vinegar. Put

everything into a pan and bring to the boil. Simmer for 10 minutes over a lower heat, Strain through a wire sieve into a basin. Discard what is left in the strainer. Pour the liquid back into the pan. Use to poach salmon.

Method: To poach fish, bring your chosen poaching liquid to the boil in a shallow pan. Lower the heat so that it simmers and put in the fish. Cod and haddock will take about 10 minutes, depending on how thick the fillets are. (Salmon steaks and fillets can be turned over after 4 minutes. Cook for another 4 minutes then test with a skewer to see if they are done) Serve hot poached fish using a fish slice to take it out of the pan and put on warm plates. If serving salmon cold, leave in the poaching liquid to cool. This will keep it moist.

Always have your vegetables and sauce almost ready before you poach fish.

Fried fish ***
Coat the fish in cornflour. Fry in hot, shallow sunflower oil, turning it over with a fish slice after 3 or 4 minutes. Serve with chips, peas and carrots.

EGGS

What a versatile, cheap and nourishing food. Eggs make a good main meal if served with hot vegetables or salad. Another bonus is they are very easy and quick to cook.

Eggs Florentine *(*1 serving) *****
Spread 1 portion of hot spinach in the centre of a warmed plate. Sprinkle with a couple of gratings of nutmeg and put a small knob of butter in the centre to melt. Top with one or two poached eggs.

Omelets

What a quick meal! Omelets can be just plain, flavoured or filled. They are not a type of food that can be kept waiting, so serve immediately. Serve with either hot steamed vegetables, a stir/stew, or with a salad.

Plain omelet (1 serving) *****

1 or 2 eggs
2 teaspoons cold water
sunflower oil for pan

Method: Break the egg(s) into a small basin and add the water. Use a fork to beat until the liquid is smooth with a little froth on top. Grease a small omelet pan with oil, using a piece of kitchen paper. When the pan is hot pour in the egg mixture. It will begin to set underneath. Break through the omelet in 3 or 4 places with a fork. Tilt the pan to let the uncooked egg run into these breaks and set. While the egg is still creamy-looking but lightly set, tip the pan away from you and loosen the edge nearest you with a knife. Fold it over on to the middle. Do the same on the other side and tip on to a warmed plate to serve immediately.

Filled omelet *****

For a filled omelet have your filling ready. When the omelet is cooked but still flat in the pan, put the filling across to one side of the the centre. Fold half the omelet over to enclose the filling. Use a fish slice to help you transfer the omelet to a warmed plate and serve immediately. Here are a few suggested fillings:

Tomato – a chopped medium tomato sprinkled with a
    teaspoon finely chopped spring onion and a teaspoon of

finely chopped fresh parsley. Garnish with a sprig of parsley.

Watercress – wash a good handful of fresh watercress sprigs and chop coarsely. Garnish with a sprig of watercress.

Mushroom – use 2 medium mushrooms, sliced finely and fried in a little sunflower oil for 2 minutes. Keep warm while you make the omelet. Garnish with a sprig of parsley.

Mixed herb – finely chop mixed fresh herbs to make a heaped teaspoon. Stir into the omelet mixture before pouring into the pan. Garnish with a sprig of parsley.

Cheese – use 1 heaped tablespoon finely grated, tasty, low fat cheddar cheese.

Cheese and tomato – use 2 heaped teaspoons finely grated, tasty, low fat cheddar cheese and 1 small tomato chopped finely

Ham – use 1 slice of ham cut into small squares. Garnish with a sprig of parsley.

Prawn – use 1 heaped tablespoon defrosted frozen prawns. Garnish with a sprig of parsley.

Salmon and cucumber – use ½ a small can of salmon and 5 or 6 thin slices cucumber, finely chopped. Garnish with a sprig of watercress or parsley.

Tuna and tomato – use ½ a small can of tuna in oil, drained, made into flakes and 1 small tomato, finely chopped. Garnish with a sprig of watercress or parsley.

Spanish omelet (2 servings) *****

2 or 3 eggs
1 teaspoon extra virgin olive oil
2 spring onions, trimmed and chopped small
1 clove garlic put through a garlic press

1½ medium sized boiled potatoes, sliced
½ red or yellow pepper, deseeded and chopped
2 heaped tablespoons cooked frozen peas
1 medium tomato, chopped small
2 teaspoons cold water
1 heaped teaspoon finely chopped fresh parsley
a few sprigs watercress or parsley for garnish

Method: Put the eggs into a small basin with the water and whisk with a fork until smooth with a little foam on the top. Heat the oil in a heavy based frying pan (not an omelet pan), add the onion and crush in the garlic. Stir/fry over a low heat for a minute. Spread the mixture over the pan. On top, arrange the potato slices and distribute the rest of the vegetables evenly. Pour the egg mixture over and cook for 30 seconds before lowering the heat. 2 or 3 minutes should be enough to set the eggs. Sprinkle with the parsley, cut the omelet in half and use a fish slice to transfer to 2 warm plates. Garnish with the parsley sprigs and serve with a crisp green salad.

Chinese style gluten-free main meal (2 or 3 servings) ****
There are no set amounts for each dish, or how many dishes there are. It all depends on how many people there are to be fed. You can get ahead by making the **sweet and sour red sauce** from chapter 8 and **crispy noodles** from chapter 3. Cut matchsticks of cooked chicken or beef and stir into the sauce. Heat through when required. Rice can be boiled in advance to be heated through (steamed in a colander with a lid on). Prepare vegetables for **stir/stew** – see chapter 6 – ready to cook at the last minute.

Rice with prawns and egg *****

boiled rice (2 – 3 heaped tablespoons before cooking)
1 tablespoon sunflower oil
4 or 5 finely chopped spring onions, including the green
1 thumb of root ginger, peeled and chopped very small
1 clove garlic put through a garlic crusher
1 egg
1 or 2 portions of cooked, defrosted prawns
handful of watercress, chopped or 6 lettuce leaves, shredded

Method: Put the rice on to reheat in a colander over a pan of boiling water. Put on a lid and steam for 5 minutes. Leave the lid on and turn out the heat. Put the oil into a saucepan and gently fry the spring onions, ginger and garlic. Break in the egg and stir with a wooden spoon to break it up as it cooks. When it starts to look dry, put in the hot rice and the prawns. Continue to heat while you fold them in. Lastly, stir in the leaves. Turn into a warm bowl and keep warm while you make the stir/stew. While you are doing this, reheat the sweet and sour sauce with the meat. (The trick is to get it all ready at the same time.) Serve it in bowls with a spoon and fork or chopsticks. The complete meal is:

rice with prawns and egg
stir/stew vegetables
sweet and sour red sauce with meat
crispy noodles
– all of which are gluten-free. Make sure you use a gluten-free soy sauce for the red sauce and stir/stew.

Savoury pancakes (makes 3) *****
Make pancakes as in chapter 3. Have ready the stuffing – 2 tablespoons plain cottage cheese, mashed, and 1 portion

chopped, cooked spinach, mixed together in a basin. Add 2 pinches grated nutmeg and season to taste. Mix and spread over the pancakes. Roll them up and keep warm until ready to serve with hot vegetables.

Pizza
See chapter 4 for pizza. Make double the recipe for a main meal and serve with a mixed or green salad. *****

Lasagne (serves 2) ****
The Bolognese sauce for this should not be too dry.

> margarine
> gluten-free pasta from chapter 3, cut into thin, rectangular sheets
> Bechamel sauce from chapter 8
> Bolognese sauce from this chapter
> finely grated Parmesan cheese or low fat tasty cheddar

Method: Grease a pie dish with margarine. Put in a spoonful of Bechamel sauce then 2 heaped tablespoons Bolognese sauce. Spread it out evenly with the back of the spoon. Cover with pasta sheets. Continue with two more layers, and end with Bechamel sauce. Sprinkle with cheese. Bake in a preheated oven at Gas 5/190° C/375° above centre shelf for about 40 minutes, until bubbling. Serve on hot plates with steamed spinach or broccoli, or, with a green side salad.

Ravioli (2 servings) *****
Little savoury parcels enclosing a tasty filling – see list below.
    Use the pasta recipe from chapter 3. Make your filling. Roll out the pasta thinly, using rice flour to dust the board. Put spoonfuls of the filling on to the pasta. Brush the pasta with cold water all round the filling using a pastry brush. Cover

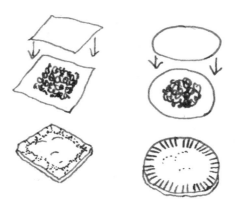

with pasta and press firmly all round the edges to seal in the filling. Go all round with the tines of a fork to make sure the edges are sealed. (If this isn't done properly the filling will leach out when they are cooked.) As you make each one, place on a plate dusted with rice flour. Have ready a large pan of boiling water. Drop in the ravioli and cook for about 5 minutes until they come to the surface. Drain in a colander and serve hot in a sauce or in vegetable broth with either a sprinkle of parsley or chopped basil leaves. See chapter 8 for Italian tomato sauce and chapter 5 for vegetable broth.

Fillings for ravioli
These should be the consistency of a paste but not be too moist. Each one is enough for filling 2 servings of ravioli.

Spinach with cheese **

½ a cup of cooked spinach, squeezed dry and chopped
1 heaped tablespoon cottage cheese, mashed
1 level tablespoon finely grated Parmesan cheese
1 tablespoon single cream
3 pinches grated nutmeg

Mix all together in a basin and use to fill ravioli. Serve cooked, in hot broth with a sprinkle of Parmesan cheese.

Mushroom *****

 1 scant tablespoon extra virgin olive oil
 ½ clove garlic put through a crusher
 1 shallot or slice of a medium onion, finely chopped
 2 medium mushrooms, finely chopped
 1 tablespoon gluten-free breadcrumbs
 1 teaspoon gluten-free soy sauce
 1 heaped teaspoon finely chopped parsley or basil
 salt and freshly ground black pepper
 1 tablespoon finely grated Parmesan cheese

Method: Fry the onion in the oil for a few seconds. Crush in the garlic and add the mushrooms. Cook for 5 minutes while you stir. Add the breadcrumbs, soy sauce, cheese and herb. Season to taste with salt and pepper. Stir well and use to fill ravioli. Serve cooked, in hot broth (see chapter 5) sprinkled with a little Parmesan cheese.

Prawns or crab ****

 2 oz (50 g) marscapone cheese
 3 oz (75g) prawns, chopped and mashed, or crabmeat
 1 teaspoon finely chopped parsley
 finely grated rind of ½ a lemon
 salt and freshly ground black pepper

Mix everything together and use to fill ravioli made with a round, fluted biscuit cutter 2½ in (6cm). Melt a little butter and mix with a squeeze of lemon juice and a teaspoon of finely chopped parsley. Pour over the ravioli to serve.

Note: Ravioli do not contain quite enough protein for a main meal. Serve after a starter of Parma ham and melon, or follow with fish or meat and a green salad.

Meat ****
Leftover Bolognese sauce (see this chapter) makes a good ravioli filling. Serve in Italian tomato sauce – see chapter 8. After draining the ravioli, put back into the pan and add a knob of margarine. Allow to coat the ravioli. This stops them sticking together before you put them into dishes. Spoon over the tomato sauce. Sprinkle with a little finely grated Parmesan before serving.

Alternatives
There are other, simpler main meals such as cold meat off a roast joint with chips/ jacket potato and salad, or bubble and squeak (see chapter 4) and gluten-free chutney.

Plain grilled meat or poultry served with chips, mashed or boiled potatoes, or boiled rice, steamed vegetables and gluten-free gravy (see chapter 8).

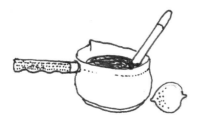

CHAPTER 8

Salad Dressings, Sauces and Gravies

Why do we need salad dressings?
The purpose of these is to moisten the salad, make it easier to eat and to enhance the flavour of the salad ingredients. Once vegetables are cut/grated they can spoil and soften. Dressing will help to slow this down. A dressing should never swamp a salad but just moisten it.

Oils, flavourings and vinegars
There are two basic kinds of salad dressing – mayonnaise and vinaigrette. Both kinds contain oil and something sharp tasting – lemon juice, one of several kinds of vinegar, garlic, onion, mustard, and herbs. The blander oils are sunflower, corn and soya. These are all fairly thin. Extra virgin olive oil is a heavier kind of oil with more flavour. Nut and seed oils such as walnut and sesame seed have a great deal of flavour. Vinegars also give a choice of flavour. Choose from wine (red

or white), cider and balsamic. Some vinegars are already flavoured with herbs. For garlic use fresh cloves. For onion use either spring onion and red onions which are not quite as fierce as the ordinary Spanish onions. One vinegar to avoid is the cheapest – malt vinegar. Always check the flavoured type.

Mustard
Mustard can be a problem. Made English mustard is usually thickened with wheat flour and is not gluten-free. However, you can buy mustard powder which just says 'mustard' on the ingredients list. This just needs mixing with a little water and is gluten-free. Genuine French mustard, made in France, is unlikely to contain wheat flour. Beware mustard made in UK or elswhere which masquerades as French mustard. It will quite likely contain wheat. Check label. Once you have found a suitable gluten-free mustard it will last you ages. (I keep a made genuine French mustard for salad dressings in the fridge and mustard powder for baking in my spice cupboard.)

SALAD DRESSINGS

The salads in chapter 6 all have suggestions for the most suitable dressings. You will need to put the vinaigrette type into a clean screw-top jar so you can give them a good shake before using, otherwise the ingredients remain separate. Stirring with a spoon has no effect.

This is the most basic of vinaigrettes with just 2 or 3 ingredients.

Oil and vinegar dressing ***
Put 3 tablespoons of sunflower oil into a small screw-top jar with 1 tablespoon of wine or cider vinegar. Put the lid on firmly. Before using, give it a good shake to combine.

For a bolder flavour add 1 level teaspoon made gluten-free mustard.

Keep shaking until the mustard has been completely absorbed by the oil and vinegar.

Oil and lemon dressing ***
Put 3 tablespoons sunflower oil into a screw-top jar with 1 tablespoon freshly squeezed lemon juice. This is a very sharp flavoured dressing so some people would prefer to add 1 level teaspoon of caster sugar. Shake before using.

Garlic dressing ***
Make the oil and vinegar dressing. Add a small, peeled clove of garlic put through a garlic press. If preferred add 1 level teaspoon caster sugar. Shake well before using. Good on green salads.

Onion dressing ***
Make the oil and vinegar dressing. Add 1 heaped teaspoon of very finely chopped onion. The white part of spring onions can be used for a mild flavour or a shallot for a stronger one. Good on mixed salads.

Mixed herb dressing ***
Make the oil and vinegar dressing. Add 2 level teaspoons finely chopped parsley and 1 teaspoon finely chopped (or snipped) chives. Good on mixed salads.

Mint dressing ***
Make the oil and vinegar dressing. Add 1 level teaspoon finely chopped fresh mint leaves. Good on new potatoes.

Chive dressing ***
Make the oil and vinegar dressing. Add 1 level teaspoon

finely chopped snipped chives. Good on green salads. Due to the intense flavours of nut oils they need to be diluted with a blander oil such as sunflower. Here are two examples.

Sesame oil dressing ***

Put 2 tablespoons of sunflower oil, 1 tablespoon of toasted sesame seed oil and 1 tablespoon of wine vinegar into a screw-top jar. Put the lid on firmly and shake well before using.

Walnut oil dressing ***

Make as for sesame seed oil dressing but substitute walnut oil for the toasted sesame seed oil.

Salad dressing – commercial style ***

As some people are hooked on this, here is a gluten-free substitute.

4 level teaspoons soya flour
1½ – 2 tablespoons wine vinegar
4 tablespoons sunflower oil
2 teaspoons caster sugar
½ level teaspoon salt
½ teaspoon gluten-free ready made mustard

Method: Put the soya flour on to a plate and press with the back of a metal spoon to get the lumps out. Put into a screw top jar with the vinegar and stir with a teaspoon. Add the oil, sugar, salt and mustard. Screw the lid on tightly and give it a good shaking to combine. Shake before using and store in the fridge.

Mayonnaise ***

There are quite a few brands of ready-made mayonnaise on the supermarket shelves. Many of them disappoint especially the light versions. Some are gluten-free. Find a suitable one you like or make your own with a liquidizer. A basic mayonnaise can be used to make several variations.

Blender mayonnaise (makes ½ pint (300ml)) ***

½ pint (300ml) sunflower oil (or extra virgin olive oil)
1 whole egg
1 egg yolk
½ level teaspoon gluten-free made mustard
2 tablespoons white wine vinegar
3 pinches salt
freshly ground black pepper
boiling water from the kettle

Method: Measure the oil into a jug. Put the egg and yolk, mustard, 1 tablespoon of the vinegar and salt into a blender. Grind in a little pepper. Put the lid on and blend for a few seconds on the lowest speed. Take out the centre cap from the lid and switch on again. Pour the oil from the jug slowly on to the blades and when the mayonnaise thickens spoon in the remaining tablespoon of vinegar and 1 tablespoon of boiling water. Spoon/scrape (with a spatula) into a clean screw-topped jar and store in the fridge for up to 2-3 weeks.

Light mayonnaise (50% less oil) (1 serving) ****
Mix 2 level tablespoons gluten-free mayonnaise with 2 level tablespoon unflavoured yoghurt. Taste. Does it need 2 pinches of caster sugar? Would a few drops of lemon juice improve it? Eat on the same day of making.

Green Mayonnaise (1 serving) to serve with cold salmon ****
Put 2 tablespoons of gluten-free light mayonnaise into a

basin. Stir in 1 teaspoon finely chopped parsley and 1 teaspoon finely chopped or snipped chives. Eat on the same day of making.

Tartare sauce (1 serving) to serve with fried fish ****
Cut a clove of garlic in half and rub it round the inside of a mixing bowl. Put in 2 tablespoons gluten-free light mayonnaise, 3 slices cucumber, finely chopped, 1 teaspoon finely chopped parsley and a small squeeze of fresh lemon juice. Mix well and eat on the day of making.

Curry mayonnaise (2 servings) to serve with cold chicken ****
Put 4 tablespoons light mayonnaise into a basin with ½ teaspoon gluten-free tomato purée, ¼ level teaspoon gluten-free mild curry powder and a few drops of fresh lemon juice. Mix well. Taste. Does it need a little more curry powder?

Pink mayonnaise (1 serving) for seafood and prawn cocktail ****
Put 2 tablespoons gluten-free light mayonnaise into a basin with 1 teaspoon gluten-free tomato purée, ¼ teaspoon caster sugar and a squeeze of lemon juice. Mix well and eat on the day of making.

SAUCES

Serving plain meat, fish and pasta would be rather boring and unappetizing without the flavour and colour of sauces. All of them can be made easily without gluten. The usual way to thicken sauces for ordinary food is with wheat flour by the roux method which can lead to much grief as it is likely to produce lumps.

For gluten-free sauces forget the dreaded roux method as

cornflour can be used instead of wheat. It is much easier to use and is not inclined to form lumps. The basis is a white sauce which can be flavoured.

Basic white sauce (makes ½ pint (300ml)) ****

    4 heaped tablespoons low-fat dried milk granules
    ½ pint (300ml) cold water
    1 level tablespoon cornflour (maize)

Method: Use a measuring jug for the water and sprinkle in the dried milk. Stir out any lumps. Put the cornflour into a cup and add 3 tablespoons of the made milk. Use a teaspoon to stir to a smooth cream. Gently heat the remaining milk in a heavy based pan. Catch it before it begins to foam and rise up. Take it off the heat and pour in the cornflour mixture while you stir. Return to a lower heat and cook/stir for 2 minutes. Don't let it boil. Use as a base for the hot savoury sauces that follow.

Parsley sauce ****
Add 1 heaped tablespoon freshly chopped parsley. Serve with grilled, baked or poached fish or boiled or roasted bacon (ham).

Watercress sauce
Add 2 heaped tablespoons freshly chopped watercress leaves. Serve with poached or baked salmon, cod, plaice and haddock.

Tomato sauce ****
Add 3 liquidised, canned, peeled plum tomatoes, 2 pinches sugar to taste and a grind of black pepper. Serve with poached, baked or grilled white fish.

Cheese sauce ***
Make as for white sauce but 1 add 1 extra level tablespoon of dried milk granules to the water. When the white sauce is made add ½ teaspoon gluten-free made mustard and a slightly rounded tablespoon of tasty, finely grated cheddar cheese. Add to the sauce but do not heat any further. Stir in until it melts. Use with white fish or to make cauliflower cheese.

Bechamel ****
Make as for white sauce but add a little grated nutmeg to taste. Use to make lasagne.

GRAVY – the most widely consumed sauce for meat and vegetables.

Brown, thick or thin and (hopefully) tasty. Dinners would be very dry without it. A *gluten-free stock* is essential. See chapter 2 for information on stock, stock cubes, gravy mixes etc.

As well as stock you will usually need a *thickener*. Cornflour or cooked potato are useful. Some gravies don't need to be thickened but beware 'watery gravy' by which every cook is judged, along with boiling an egg. Gravy made with wheat flour is prone to lumps. This problem is less likely with a gluten-free thickener. Try not to serve the same gravy whatever the food as this is boring and doesn't stimulate the appetite. Here are some suggestions to avoid this.

Basic gravy (1 serving) – a base for adding appropriate flavouring. ****

    1 level teaspoon cornflour mixed with 2 tablespoons cold
        water
    1 teaspoon gluten-free soy sauce (or other gluten-free stock)
    about ¾ cup of water.

Method: Mix and pour into a small pan. Bring to the boil then lower heat and simmer for a minute while you stir. For thin gravy use a little less cornflour, for a thicker gravy use a little more.

For a thick gravy you can add a teaspoon of mashed potato, but don't overdo it as it will make the texture gluey.

Flavourings
Don't let a flavoured gravy overwhelm the meal. It should merely enhance the flavours of the meat and vegetables, not be the main flavour. It should relate to the food on the plate not clash with it.

- If you have saved vegetable strainings from the meal you have cooked, these can be used instead of water.
- *Meat Juices.* These can be found in the grill pan and roasting tin. Alas they also come with the meat fat and require putting through a gravy separator. This simple piece of kitchen kit is a jug with two spouts. One spout is at the top like an ordinary jug and the other comes from right down the bottom. The fat separates out from the meat juices and rises to the top, enabling the meat juices to be poured off from the bottom to make the gravy. Empty the grill pan or roasting tin into the separator and let it settle for a minute. Pour out the juices into the basic gravy and heat before serving.
- *Mustard* – Add ¼ level teaspoon of made gluten-free mustard if serving with beef or just to perk up an otherwise dull gravy.
- *Tomato* – Add ½ level teaspoon tomato purée. This adds to the colour as well as the taste. Good for vegetarian burgers, roasts as well as meat burgers
- *Onion* – Fry a small piece of very finely chopped fresh

onion in 2 teaspoons sunflower oil and add to the gravy
before bringing to the boil.
* *Herbs* – finely chop a fresh herb or mixture of herbs
  appropriate for the meat in the meal. Enough to make a
  good pinch will do. If using dried versions a small pinch
  will be enough to flavour the gravy.

If serving to the whole family just multiply up the ingredients.
Gluten-free gravy can be just as good if not better than ordi-
nary gravy thickened with wheat flour.
   Note*: Your stock and thickener must be gluten-free.*

Sweet and sour red sauce (4 servings) ***
A sauce to use for Chinese style meals or stir/stew.

   1 level tablespoon cornflour
   2 tablespoons wine vinegar
   1 tablespoon sugar
   juice of 1 medium orange
   ½ pint (300ml) cold water
   1 tablespoon sunflower oil
   1 heaped teaspoon finely chopped root ginger
   1 clove garlic put through a crusher
   2 spring onions, trimmed and chopped finely, including the
      green stalks
   1 level tablespoon tomato purée
   1½ tablespoons gluten-free soy sauce

Method: Put the cornflour into a basin with the vinegar, sugar
and orange juice. Mix well and add the water. In a small pan
gently fry the ginger, garlic and spring onions in the sunflower oil while you stir for a minute. Pour in the mixture
from the basin and bring gently to the boil, still stirring. When
it has thickened, stir in the tomato purée and soy sauce. Serve

hot with Chinese style food to all the family. See chapter 3 for crispy noodles and chapter 7 for a Chinese meal.

Fresh Mint Sauce *(2-3 servings (cold))* ***

1 handful fresh mint leaves – about 6 stems
3 teaspoons wine vinegar
2 slightly heaped teaspoons caster sugar
1 tablespoon boiling water from the kettle

Method: Wash the mint. Pull off the leaves and discard the stalks. Put on to a board and chop finely with a large, sharp knife. Spoon into a small bowl and stir in the sugar in with a teaspoon. Add the boiling water and stir until the sugar has dissolved. Lastly, add the vinegar and stir in. Traditionally served with roast or grilled lamb.

Apple sauce (2-3 servings) ****
This sauce should not be sweet. It needs to be tart.

1 medium cooking apple, peeled, cored and sliced thinly
the cut off end of 1 lemon
about 2 tablespoons water
2 teaspoons caster sugar
small knob of margarine

Method: Put the apple, lemon and water into a small pan. Cover and cook gently for about 10 minutes, until the apple is soft. Take off the heat and remove and discard the lemon. Stir in the sugar and beat to a purée. Serve with roast pork, duck or vegetarian roast.

St.Clements BBQ sauce – makes about ¾ pint (450 ml) ***
Everyone will like to share this gluten-free sauce.

1 medium onion, finely chopped
1 oz (25g) polyunsaturated soft margarine
2 oz (50g) soft brown sugar
1 level tablespoon cornflour
2 teaspoon gluten-free made mustard
1 teaspoon gluten-free soy sauce
finely grated rind of ½ and orange
juice of 1 orange and 1 lemon
1 level tablespoon tomato purée
½ pint (300ml) water
salt and freshly ground black pepper to taste

Method: Use a medium pan to gently cook the onion in the
margarine for about 10 minutes, stirring from time to time.
Mix the cornflour with 2 tablespoons cold water in a basin.
Put in the remaining ingredients and mix well, getting out
any lumps. Add to the onions and bring to the boil, stirring
all the time. Reduce heat to simmer for 5 minutes. Taste and
adjust seasoning. Serve with grilled or barbequed chicken
and beef.

Pesto (2 – 3 servings) ****
Use on gluten-free pasta. See recipe in chapter 7.

About 2 oz (50g) handful of fresh basil leaves
1 pinch salt
3 grinds black pepper
1 clove garlic, put through a crusher
3 tablespoons extra virgin olive oil
1 oz (25g) pine nuts or walnuts (optional)
2 level tablespoons finely grated Parmesan cheese

Method: Put all ingredients into a small food processor and
blend to a smooth paste. Alternatively, put ingredients into a

mortar and pound with a pestle, but adding the oil a few drops at a time.

Italian tomato sauce (makes ½ pint (300ml)) ****
This sauce thickens itself as it cooks. If it thickens too much you may need to add a little hot water.

1 tablespoon extra virgin olive oil
½ a medium onion, finely chopped
1 medium can chopped, peeled plum tomatoes
1 medium carrot, finely grated
1 slick celery, sliced thinly
2 level teaspoons tomato purée
1 teaspoon caster sugar
1 clove garlic put through a crusher
salt and freshly ground black pepper to taste
about 8 leaves fresh basil, finely chopped, or 1 level
    teaspoon dried

Method: Put the first 8 ingredients into a medium sized saucepan. Stir and bring to the boil. Partially cover the pan (to let the steam out) and reduce heat to simmer for about 30 minutes. Allow to cool for a few minutes then liquidize. Add salt and pepper to taste and stir in the basil. Serve with pasta, as part of a pizza or with chicken or fish.

TABLE SAUCES

Tomato Ketchup ****
An all-round and very popular table sauce. Good with breakfasts, eggs, fish, burgers, fishcakes etc. The commercial version of this is sold in infuriating sauce bottles, either glass or squeezy plastic. A jam jar with a screw on lid can be used for the home made version. Store in the fridge with the lid on.

1 medium tin peeled plum tomatoes, chopped
2 teaspoons tarragon flavoured vinegar
2 heaped teaspoons soft brown sugar
2 pinches each of cinnamon, cayenne pepper, ground mace
     and allspice
1 tablespoon water

Method: Put all ingredients into a saucepan. Bring to the boil then lower the heat and simmer until it has reduced to a thick sauce. (Give it a stir from time to time.) Cool a little then liquidize in a blender. Taste. Does it need a pinch or two of salt? Spoon into a sterilized jar with a lid. Store in the fridge.

Note. If you don't feel it tastes strong enough, stir in a teaspoon of tomato purée.

Here is another table sauce, the brown, fruit version of tomato ketchup.

Brown fruit sauce – rich, spicy and fruity for the table. Keeps well. ****

3 oz (75g) dates, stoned and chopped
3 oz (75g) chopped tomato
6 oz (185g) cooking apple, peeled and chopped
2 oz (50g) onion, peeled and chopped
4 fluid oz (125 ml) wine vinegar
1 tablespoon fresh lemon juice
6 fluid oz (190 ml) water
½ clove garlic, put through a crusher
2 teaspoon gluten-free soy sauce (see note below)
3 good pinches ground ginger
2 good pinches ground cloves
¼ teaspoon salt
2 slightly heaped teaspoons brown sugar

Method: Have ready a sterilized jar and lid. Put the dates, tomatoes, apple and onion into a saucepan with the vinegar. Cook while stirring for 5 or 6 minutes until soft. Add the lemon juice and water. Blend in a liquidizer and return to pan. Crush in the garlic and spoon in the soy sauce, spices, salt and sugar. Stir and bring to the boil. Lower heat and simmer while you stir to reduce it – about 3 or 4 minutes should be enough. Put through a wire sieve into a basin to remove pips and tomato skins. Put back into the pan and bring to the boil again. Pour into the prepared jar and put the lid on. When cool, store in the fridge.

Note: The soy sauce must be gluten-free – Tamari type (not brand) – made on a rice base instead of wheat. Check label before using.

SWEET SAUCES

These are for puddings and desserts, both hot and cold. Probably the most popular is custard, one of the first allergy foods from the nineteenth century. At that time custard was made with just eggs, which didn't agree with those allergic to them.

The substitute is still going strong in the form of vanilla flavoured cornflour with a natural yellow colouring. It is served on fruit pies, crumbles, stewed fruit, tarts and all kinds of hot puddings. You can buy ready-made custard in tins and cartons but they are not necessarily gluten-free, so check before using. Alternatively make your own at home. If you don't have a commercial brand of custard powder, use cornflour and add a few drops of vanilla flavouring.

However, it won't be yellow, it will be white. All cornflour based custards will form a skin as they grow cold, A piece of greaseproof paper on the top of the actual custard will stop a skin forming. Custard takes longer to cook in the microwave than it does on the hob. (A non-stick pan is ideal for making custard and kind to the person washing up.)

Custard (makes ½ pint (300ml)) to serve hot ***

> 1 level tablespoon gluten-free custard powder (check label)
> 1 level tablespoon sugar
> ½ pint (300ml) skimmed milk

Method: Put the custard powder into a basin with the sugar and two tablespoons of the milk. Heat the remaining milk in a pan until nearly boiled. Catch it before it begins to foam and rise up. Pour on to the custard mix while you stir. Return to the pan and heat to boiling point, stirring gently all the time. Serve hot on hot puddings.

Chocolate sauce *(*makes ½ pint (300ml)) ***
Make as for custard but add 2 heaped teaspoons cocoa to the basin before mixing. Serve on hot chocolate sponge pudding.

Orange or lemon sauce ****
Make as for custard but use cornflour instead of custard powder. Add the rind of ½ grated orange or lemon, stirred into the finished sauce.

Melba sauce *(*makes 1 portion) ***
Prepare a handful each of raspberries and redcurrants. Stew in a little water until soft. Cool for 5 minutes then put into a mini food processor. Blend to a purée then put through a wire mesh sieve into a bowl. Use a wooden spoon to press it through. Sweeten to taste with caster sugar. Use with gluten-free sponge and custard.

Raspberry sauce ****
If you only have a few, mash raspberries on a plate. If you have a quantity, put into the liquidizer with a little water and blend. Put through a wire mesh sieve to remove the pips, catching the juice in a basin. Sweeten to taste and use with fresh fruit. See recipe in chapter 9 for Fruit Plate.

Chocolate sauce for profiteroles – liquid chocolate **

 2 oz (50 g) dark gluten-free cooking chocolate
 water
 1 level teaspoon instant coffee granules
 3 oz (75g) caster sugar

Method: Dissolve the coffee granules in 2 teaspoons water. Break the chocolate into pieces and put into a small pan with 4 tablespoons water. Heat very gently to melt the chocolate. Add the coffee liquid and sugar. Continue over a gentle heat while you stir for another few minutes. Leave to cool. Heat again when required to pour hot over profiteroles or ice cream.

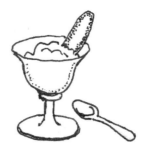

CHAPTER 9

Fruit, Puddings and Desserts

All fresh and frozen plain fruit is gluten-free. As we should all be eating 3 pieces of fruit per day, more of an interest in fruit would seem to be a good gluten-free idea. Because fruit salad is easy to make it tends to be neglected. With the variety of fresh fruit in supermarkets all year round, fruit salad can be a treasure house of delight. A combination of banana, apple and orange can seem quite boring but pineapple, papaya and passion fruit give fruit salad a different dimension. Here is a typical list of fresh and frozen fruit from which to choose:

apples, pears, bananas, seedless grapes
mango, papaya, kiwi fruit
   strawberries, raspberries, cherries
blackcurrants, blackberries, blueberries
apricots, peaches, nectarines, dessert plums
oranges, clementines

redcurrants, fruits of the forest (mixtures)
melons, lychees, passion fruit

(I have deliberately left off grapefruit as many people with digestion problems have a problem with it, also rhubarb and damson because they are so sour and require a lot of sugar.)

Fruit salad *****
Try to make it colourful. Don't put several pale fruits together e.g. melon, apple pear and banana. It will just look washed out. On the other hand, coloured fruits are always more exciting and can be used to make a contrast with the paler colours. Some fruits can look quite dramatic in a fruit salad. Blueberries, black cherries and kiwi fruit, redcurrants, raspberries and strawberries will perk up any combination.

In any fruit salad you will need some kind of juice or it will be too dry and start to turn brown. If you buy ripe fruit it should be sweet enough as it is. To be refreshing it can be a little tart. Forget the high sugar levels of cakes, chocolate bars and sweets. These are man-made. The sweetness of fruit is just natural. However, a *little* sugar is in order if the fruit is too sharp and sour.

As soon as you cut up fruit it begins to deteriorate, so don't make a fruit salad until just before you need it. Basically, have a look at what is in the fruit bowl and select four or five pieces of ripe fruit, one of which should be a bright colour. Wash, peel and cut them into bite -sized pieces. Put into a bowl, add fruit juice to moisten and a little caster sugar only if necessary. If you cut the fruit into small pieces you can call it 'fruit cocktail'. If you only buy fruit in season you will enjoy fruit salads that are different throughout the year and they will be less expensive.

One fruit that is nothing to look at but is guaranteed to lift any combination of fruit is passion fruit. Cut in half and take out the inside with a teaspoon. Put into the bowl, seeds and all. Lychees also have a great effect but they are white and so don't have much visual impact. However, they taste very exotic. Papaya, mango, and pineapple are also exotic and have a strong taste compared to apples and pears. Cut them into small pieces.

Fruit plate with raspberry juice (serves 1) *****

This is the most colourful, show-off dessert possible for a gluten-free dieter to eat when everyone else is having something with wheat. It is very simple and very easy to make, looking stunning when served on a plain white plate. You will need five kinds of fruit,in small amounts, one of which should be melon. To make the raspberry juice, blitz a handful of fresh raspberries in a small food processor. Put through a sieve over a basin to make the brilliant red juice. Sweeten to taste with caster sugar. Arrange the fruit in groups, so it will lie flat on the plate and arrange it so the colours complement each other. A typical arrangement would be 2 long slices of melon, 4 slices of peeled kiwi fruit, 3 halved strawberries, about 5 raspberries and 6 or 7 blueberries. Put the juice into a little jug. Pour it carefully in the centre of the plate so it spreads around the fruit and not over it.

Serve with a small knife and fork and wait for the envious

looks. Other fruits to use are peeled papaya, cut in long thin slices, 2 long slices of peeled mango and 5 small pieces of fresh pineapple. Avoid apple, pear and banana as they will discolour.

Fresh fruit *****
The simplest of all puddings is a piece of fresh fruit, ripe, sweet, good quality, nicely prepared and presented. Choose one from the following:

Orange, – peeled and the segments separated and made into a wheel on a white plate.

Clementine – allow 2 and present as for orange

Papaya – cut in half lengthways, remove pips with a teaspoon. Cut a small flat slice from the skin at the back for it to balance on. Shaped avocado dishes are ideal for serving this attractive and scented fruit.

Pear – peel, core and quarter. Cut lengthways into slices and arrange in a fan, slightly overlapping. Eat soon after preparing.

Strawberry – hull and halve. Arrange in a circle.

Raspberries – arrange in a small heap in a dish.

Dessert apple such as 'Pink Lady' – peel, core and slice. Arrange overlapping, in a circle. Unless served immediately it will begin to turn brown.

Peach – rub all over with the flat of a knife. Cut in half and remove stone. Peel then cut into slices and arrange in a fan shape.

Nectarine – halve and remove stone, arrange as for a peach.

Kiwi fruit – cut in half around the middle, don't peel. Serve with a teaspoon and eat as you would a boiled egg.

Pineapple – Cut off the top and bottom then the tough

skin. Quarter the fruit lengthways. Cut out the central
fibrous core from each quarter. Slice then cut into
pieces. Make a small pile in a dish.
Melon – Cut in half. Scoop out and discard the seeds with
a spoon. Cut into halves again and with a sharp,pointed
knife, cut away the flesh from the hard skin. Either cut
into long, thin slices and arrange in a fan, overlapping,
on a plate, to eat with a knife and fork, or, cut into
cubes and put into a dish with a teaspoon.
Lychees – Pull away the hard, outer casing. Slice the flesh
away from the centre seed. Serve in a small glass dish
with a teaspoon.
Mango – eaten on its own this fruit can be very laxative.
For this reason it is usually combined with another
fruit, in small amounts. Peel the fruit and slice away the
flesh from the stone. (In my house mango is known as
'paint stripper'.)

See also chapter 12 for **fruit kebabs**

Stewed fruit ****
Pick ripe, fresh stewing fruit – cooking apples, pears, plums,
apricots, greengages, black and red currants, raspberries,
blackcurrant, blackberries etc. Frozen fruit is available all
year round. Fruits of the forest mixtures and summer berries
are good buys as they can be used with stewed apple. Old
favourites are blackberry and apple and just stewed apple on
its own. Some fruits are good baked in the oven on their
own – apricots, cooking apples and pears. Just make sure
you have enough water in the dish. Bake on the centre shelf
in a pie dish. Peel pears but leave the skin on cooking apples
and cut a ring all round as well as taking out the core. (If
you don't do this they are inclined to burst.) For apricots,
plums and greengages make a slit in the natural join. Bake

whole with the stones still in. Bake until tender on any temperature. Apples can be stuffed with gluten-free mincemeat in the centre. Pears can be baked with a tablespoon of summerfruits in the water. This will tint the pears a pretty lavender colour.

Fruit snow (serves 2) ****
This is the lightest of desserts as there is no fat in it.

  1 medium Bramley cooking apple
  1 heaped tablespoon fresh or frozen raspberries
  1 tablespoon water
  1 medium egg white
  1 level tablespoon of caster sugar

Method: Peel and core the apple. Cut into thin slices and put into a pan with the raspberries and water Cook over a gentle heat with the lid on until soft. Beat with a wooden spoon or put through a small food processor to make a smooth purée. Allow to cool. Put the egg white into a small basin and beat with a hand beater until stiff and forming peaks. Sprinkle in the sugar and whisk until it begins to look shiny. Fold into the fruit purée with a metal spoon and divide between two glasses. Put into the fridge and serve cold. Very light and refreshing.

  Note: Other fruit can be used instead of raspberries such as blackberries, and black or red currants. Apple can be used on its own with the grated rind of ¼ of a lemon.

Real fruit jelly ****
Most fruit can be used for jelly but not the more exotic such as pineapple and kiwi as these contain an enzyme called bromelain. This is a protein digesting enzyme. It gets to work on the gelatin and stops the jelly from setting.

The method is the same for all the following flavours. The recipe is for about 3 or 4 portions. The fruit juice can be made from blending fresh fruit in a liquidizer or from stewing fruit in water or a combination of both.

1 pint (550 ml) fruit juice
caster sugar to taste
1 x ½ oz (15g) sachet gelatin

Method: Put 4 tablespoons of the fruit juice into a cup. Sprinkle the gelatin slowly into this and leave for it to soften for about 5 minutes. While you are waiting, put the remainder of the fruit juice into a saucepan and heat to *almost* boiling point. Add sugar to taste and stir to dissolve. Pour into a basin or 3 or 4 glass dishes and allow to cool. Put in the fridge and don't move it for at least 2 hours while it sets. Serve straight from the fridge and eat within 24 hours.

Suggested fruit combinations follow to make 1 pint (550ml) of juice which can be put through a strainer to remove pips etc., or made up with water. Pieces of fresh fruit can be put into the bottom of the basin or glasses and the jelly poured over.

Raspberry and orange – ½ lb (¼ kilo) fresh raspberries and orange juice.
Strawberry and orange – ½ lb (¼ kilo) hulled strawberries and orange juice.
Peach and strawberry – 2 stoned peaches and a handful of hulled strawberries.
Peach melba – 2 stoned peaches, raspberries and red currants (strain through a sieve.)
Summerfruits – juice made by stewing 1 pack of frozen summerfruits in a little water.

Steamed fruit pudding (serves 4) ****
This is very similar in taste, texture and appearance to wheat
flour suet pastry yet it is gluten-free. A hearty, warm-you-up
winter pudding to serve to all the family. You will need a 1
pint (550ml) heatproof pudding basin with a lid.

> 2 oz (50g) polyunsaturated soft margarine
> 4 oz (100g) ground rice
> 3 oz (75g) eating apple, finely grated
> stewing fruit for the filling (raw) – just over ½ lb (¼ kilo)
>   after preparing – see note below
> granulated sugar to taste, about 2 tablespoons
> 1 tablespoon water
> rice flour for kneading etc.

Grease the pudding basin and put a large pan on to boil,
full of water. Place a metal grid or 3 metal forks in the
bottom. Put the margarine into a bowl with the ground rice
and grated apple. Blend with a fork into a stiff paste. Knead
by hand into 1 ball using a little more rice flour if it is too
wet. Roll of the pastry into a ball and flatten. Place this in
the bottom of the basin. Press with your fingers to spread it
up the sides of the basin, stopping at ½ inch (1¼ cm) below
the rim.

Make the remaining of the pastry into a flat circle, on a
piece of food film, either by hand or with a rolling pin. Put
half the prepared fruit into the basin and sprinkle with sugar.
Add the rest and sprinkle again. Pour in the water and put on
the pastry lid by turning it upside down and peeling it off the
food film. Press all round to join the lid to the sides. Put on
the lid of the basin and lower the pudding into the pan of boiling water. Make sure the forks or the grid come between the
bottom of the basin and the pan. Put on the saucepan lid and
steam for about 45 minutes. Watch the water level does not go

down. If it does, top up with more boiling water from the kettle. When it is done, take the basin out of the saucepan and remove the lid. Cover the pudding with a plate, hold them firmly together and turn upside down. Leave on the worktop for a few seconds for the pudding to drop on to the plate. Carefully shake and remove the basin. Serve hot with gluten-free custard.

Fruit: For the filling use apple, blackberry and apple, apricots, greengages, peaches, cooking pears, plums, apple and summer fruits (defrosted), any mixture in season or frozen defrosted.

Soufflé omelet (serves 1) ****
A high protein pudding to make quickly, as required.

  2 medium eggs, separated
  1 tablespoon single cream
  2 teaspoons caster sugar
  small knob of margarine
  1 generous tablespoon jam or stewed fruit such as
      blackberries (sweetened)
  icing sugar for finishing

Method: Separate the egg yolks and whites. Put the egg yolks into a basin with the cream and beat well with a hand whisk. In a separate basin, whisk the egg whites until stiff and fold (don't beat) them into the yolk mixture, with a metal spoon. Melt the margarine in an omelet pan and pour in the soufflé mixture. Spread out evenly and lightly with the back of the spoon. Cook over a medium heat for a minute until browning underneath. Take off the hob and put under a hot grill until the top has set. Heat the jam in a small pan and spread over half the omelet. Use a palette knife to fold the plain half over. Dust with icing sugar, using a sieve. Serve hot immediately.

Note: For a more exciting way to serve a souffle omelet, see chapter 12.

Pear and chocolate pudding (serves 3 or 4) ***

    2 ripe pears, peeled, cored and sliced thinly
    1 tablespoon soft brown sugar (optional)
    chocolate flavoured sponge mixture from chapter 10

Method: Preheat oven at Gas 4/180° C/350 °F. Peel and core pears. Cut into slices and place in a greased, shallow oven-proof dish. Make the chocolate sponge mixture and spread over the pears. Bake for about 25 minutes and test with a skewer. If it comes out clean it is baked. Serve out of the dish, warm or cold, with single cream or custard if warm and unflavoured set yoghurt if cold.

Note: If the pears are very sweet you will not need the sugar.

Eve's pudding (serves 3 or 4) ***
Make as for pear and chocolate pudding but omit pears and use cooking apples instead, slicing them thinly. Omit cocoa from the sponge mixture.

Pancakes (makes 3) ****
See chapter 3 for batter recipe and how to make them.

The classic way to serve these is with lemon juice and caster sugar. Make the pancakes, squeeze over a little lemon juice and sprinkle with caster sugar. Roll up each one and serve hot on a warm plate with a little sprinkle of sugar.

Fruit pancakes (serves 2) ****
Make the pancakes as in chapter 3 and keep warm. Have ready about 6 tablespoons stewed fruit, sweetened to taste.

Put 1 pancake on to a warm, greased ovenproof plate and spread 3 tablespoons stewed fruit over it. Put another pancake on top and repeat, ending with a pancake. Serve warm, cut into wedges. Alternatively, spread filling over each one and roll up. Finish with a sprinkle of caster sugar. Choose one of the following for the stewed fruit:

apple with a teaspoon finely grated lemon rind
blackberry and apple
apple and raspberry
apple and blackcurrants
apple, 3 pinches cinnamon and 1 tablespoon sultanas
apple and summer fruits
fresh apricots
plums and damsons
rhubarb

Crêpes Suzette (serves 2) ***
Make pancakes as directed in chapter 3 but make 4 pancakes instead of 3. Keep warm, stacked on a plate, one on top of the other, under a clean tea towel

1 oz (25g) margarine
1oz (25g) caster sugar
finely grated rind and juice of 1 orange

Method: Put a serving dish to warm. Melt the margarine in a frying pan. Add the sugar, orange rind and juice. Stir and heat until it bubbles. Dip each pancake into the sauce, fold in half, then in half again. Put into the warmed dish, pour the rest of the hot sauce over and serve immediately, on warm plates.

Note: For a much more spectacular way of serving these, see chapter 12.

Hot chocolate pudding (serves 1) ***
This is really quick and easy to make, especially nice on a
cold winter's day.

2 level tablespoons rice flour
2 level tablespoons dried low fat milk powder
1 tablespoon caster sugar
4 drops vanilla flavouring
3 level teaspoons cocoa
about 7 fluid oz (200ml) water

Method: Stir the milk powder into the water until dissolved.
Mix the rice flour with the cocoa in a small basin. Add a little
of the milk and stir to make a cream. Add more milk and stir
again. Turn into the remaining milk. Put in the vanilla flavouring and sugar. Mix well, pour into a small pan and heat gently
while stirring. Bring to the boil, still stirring, then lower heat
and simmer for 3 minutes or until thickened. Serve hot in a
bowl.

Fruit crumble (2 servings) ***

2 portions stewed fruit, sweetened to taste
2 teaspoons ground almonds
2 generous tablespoons ground rice
1 tablespoon sunflower oil
1 oz (25g) demerara sugar

Method: Preheat the oven at Gas 7/220 °C/425 °F. Put the
stewed fruit into an ovenproof dish and flatten the top
evenly. Put the ground almonds into a bowl with the ground
rice and mix well. Rub in the oil until the mixture resembles
crumbs. Stir in the sugar. Spoon over the stewed fruit and
make a hole through to the fruit in the centre to let out the

steam. Bake for 10 minutes on the top shelf. Serve hot or cold.

Cooked fresh or dried fruits are suitable for the base – dried apricots, prunes or apricots, plums, gooseberries, black-currant and apple, apple with a little finely grated lemon rind, stewing pears, rhubarb etc.

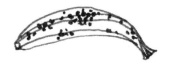

Author's Erratum

I apologize for the following mistake in the recipe for Shortbread on page 147. The ingredients list should read 2oz (50g) of the flour blend and 1 level tablespoon of the jam – sugar with pectin.

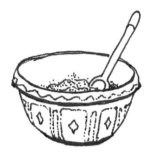

CHAPTER 10

Cakes, Biscuits, Cookies, Pastries

This chapter is for everyday food. (Chapter 12 has the over-the-top celebration food). On a gluten-free diet is very easy to concentrate too much on sugary cakes and biscuits to the exclusion of fruit and vegetables. Try not to eat too many sweet things out of habit. Here is a selection of easy to make items with a variety of flavours to choose from. Easiest to start with is the shortbread and fruit sponge buns or fairy cakes.

Shortbread (makes 4 or 6 crisp and golden biscuits) ***

    1 oz (25g) polyunsaturated soft margarine
    pinch of salt
    ½ oz (25g) RG77 gluten-free flour blend (see chapter 3)
    1½ oz (15g) jam – sugar with pectin (see chapter 3)
    3 drops vanilla flavouring
    2 teaspoons cold water

Method: Preheat oven at Gas 3/160° C/325° F. Grease a baking sheet. Put the flour into a mixing bowl with the salt. Mix. Add the margarine and rub in with the fingertips until the mixture resembles crumbs. Sprinkle in the sugar. Mix, then put in the vanilla flavouring and 2 teaspoons cold water. Mix together by hand to form one ball of dough. Knead for just 30 seconds and put on to the prepared baking sheet. Spread out with your fingers into a circle about 5 inches (13 cm) in diameter. Pinch up the edges all round and press in the tines of a fork to make a pattern. Cut with a knife to make 4 or 6 wedges. Bake on the centre shelf for about 30 minutes. Leave on the baking sheet for 2 minutes before taking them off with a spatula. Put on a wire rack to cool. When cold, wrap individually in food film and store in an airtight container. Eat within 5 days.

Whisked sponge (low fat,makes 6-8 slices) ****
This is a very light, quickly baked sponge that can be dressed up for an occasion. It needs to be eaten freshly made as it doesn't stay fresh for long, having very little fat in it. As there are 3 eggs it does not need baking powder.You will need 2 small, round sponge tins 6 in (5cm). If you have an electric beater you won't need the pan of hot water.

4 oz (100g) RG77 gluten-free flour blend
4 pinches Xanthan gum
3 medium eggs
4½ oz (125g) caster sugar
4 drops vanilla flavouring

Method: Grease the edges and line the bases of 2 sponge tins 6in (15cm) with baking parchment. Preheat oven at Gas 5/190°C/375°F. Mix the flour and Xanthan gum in a basin. Arrange a bowl over a pan of hot water. Put in the eggs, sugar and flavouring and whisk with a hand whisk until very thick.

Fold in the flour mixture. (Don't beat or you will knock the air out of it.) Pour into the prepared tins. Bake for about 20 minutes on the centre shelf of the oven. The sponges should spring back when lightly pressed with a finger if they are done. Leave in the tins for 5 minutes to allow them to shrink round the edges. (You can run a knife around to make sure they will release.) Turn upside down on to a wire rack and remove papers. When cold, sandwich together with jam and sprinkle the top with icing sugar.

Note: Don't overbake these delicate sponges. They should be pale golden brown. See chapter 12 for how to dress them up as a gateau for a party. They can also be used for dessert – see chapter 9 – and any stale sponge can be used for trifle.

Fairy cakes (makes 6) light as a feather, easy to make, enviable little buns. ***
Nobody will know they are gluten-free until you tell them and they come in eight flavours. (They are too light for dried fruit etc.) You will need a shallow patty tin and cake papers.

2½oz (65g) RG77 gluten-free flour blend (see chapter 3)
2 pinches Xanthan gum
¾ level teaspoon gluten-free baking powder
2 oz (50g) polyunsaturated soft margarine
1 medium egg
2 oz (50g) caster sugar
flavouring of your choice – see list below

Method: Preheat oven at Gas 5/190°/375°. Line a patty tin with 6 cake papers. Put the flour, Xanthan gum, baking powder, margarine, egg and sugar into a bowl. Mix then beat to a cream using a wooden spoon. Add the flavouring of your choice and mix again. Spoon into the cake papers and bake on the top shelf for about 15 minutes. When pressed with a finger the buns should spring back. Cool on a wire rack. Best eaten freshly baked. When cold, wrap individually in food film.

Flavours: (choose just *one* from the list)
Orange – finely grated rind of ¼ of an orange
Lemon – finely grated rind of ¼ lemon
Ginger – ½ level teaspoon ground ginger
Chocolate – 1 heaped teaspoon cocoa and 1 teaspoon water
Coffee – mix 1 level teaspoon of instant coffee with 1 teaspoon water
Spice – 1 level teaspoon mixed spice
Cinnamon – ½ level teaspoon cinnamon
Vanilla – 6 drops vanilla flavouring

Fruit sponge buns (makes 6) ****
These delightful little buns are baked in paper cases and between them will hold up 1 oz (25g) of dried fruit but no more, as they are soft and light. (Nobody will suspect they are gluten free). Ideally, eat while they are still warm for tea, or elevenses or a lunchbox treat. Just double the recipe to make a dozen for the whole family. The binder is in the jam sugar which contains pectin (made from fruit.) You can add ground almonds if you wish as this will make them keep fresh for longer.

As always, check before using dried fruit. Some will have added sugar made from wheat –– 'wheat fructose- sucrose' or similar – and should not be used. Glacé cherries and candied peel need special attention. The syrup on glacé cherries may contain gluten from wheat. You will need to shop around for gluten-free versions. Try health stores. See chapter 2.

Measure exactly. Don't guess and avoid disaster.

¾ level teaspoon gluten-free baking powder (use a ½
  teaspoon and a ¼ teaspoon to measure or 3 x ¼
  teaspoons)
2½ oz (65g) RG77 gluten-free flour blend (see chapter 3)
1 medium egg
2 oz (50g) polyunsaturated soft margarine
1 level tablespoon ground almonds (optional)
1½ oz (40g) jam-sugar with pectin
flavouring/fruit of your choice – see list below

Method: Preheat oven at Gas 5/190°C/375°F. Line a patty tin
with 6 cake papers. Put the first six ingredients into a bowl
and mix/beat to a creamy consistency. Stir in the fruit/flavour-
ing of your choice. Divide equally between the paper cases
and bake on the top shelf for about 12 minutes or until well
risen and golden. When pressed with a finger they will spring
back if they are done. Leave in the tin for about 3 minutes
then transfer to a wire rack to cool. When cold, wrap individually in food film. Eat within two days.

Fruit and flavourings for fruit sponge buns:

- *Currants* – add 1 oz (25g) currants and finely grated
  rind of ¼ of a lemon.
- *Sultanas* – add 1 oz (25g) sultanas and finely grated rind
  of ¼ of a lemon or orange.
- *Raisins* – add 1 oz (25g) raisins and finely grated rind of
  ¼ of an orange
- *Mixed fruit* – make your own mixture with currants,
  sultanas and chopped dried apricots. They should total
  1 oz (25g). Add with finely grated rind of ¼ of a
  lemon.
- *Apricot* – add 5 dried apricots, chopped and ½ level
  teaspoon cinnamon.

- *Seed* – add 1 slightly heaped teaspoon caraway seeds.
- *Coconut* – add 1 slightly heaped tablespoon dessicated coconut. Make 7 instead of 6.
- *Blueberries* – add 1 slightly heaped tablespoon dried blueberries.
- *Coffee and walnut* – add 3 finely chopped walnut halves and 1 teaspoon instant coffee dissolved in 1 teaspoon water.
- *Chocolate* – add 5 drops vanilla flavouring and 1 heaped teaspoon cocoa.
- *Chocolate and hazelnut* – add 5 drops of vanilla flavouring, 1 heaped teaspoon cocoa and 1 heaped tablespoon chopped, toasted hazelnuts.
- *Date and ginger* – add 3 chopped, stoned dates and ½ level teaspoon dried ginger.
- *Marmalade* – add just the orange peel from marmalade, enough to make ½ oz (15g)

Fresh fruit additions
These buns will take 1 oz (25g) fresh fruit if chopped small. Stoned cherries, pineapple, peach, and strawberry, all with 5 drops vanilla flavouring; eating apple or plum with ½ teaspoon cinnamon or mixed spice; pear with 1 level teaspoon cocoa. Eat freshly baked.

Quick golden sponge (makes 4 slices) from 1 sponge ***
This recipe has a curious characteristic. If baked on a higher heat (Gas 5/190°C/375°F) it will rise well but at the base of each sponge will be a paler layer. It doesn't alter the flavour but it looks interesting if the sponge is sandwiched with a dark coloured jam. If you don't want this effect, bake at Gas 4/180°C/350°F.

2½ oz (65g) RG77 gluten free flour blend (see chapter 3)
¾ level teaspoon gluten-free baking powder
2 oz (50g) polyunsaturated soft margarine
2 oz (50g) caster sugar
1 medium egg
few drops vanilla flavouring

Method: Preheat oven at Gas 5/190°C/375°F. Line a 6 in (15cm) round sponge tin with baking parchment. (Cut it larger than the tin then snip all the way round.) Put all ingredients into a bowl and mix/beat with a wooden spoon, to a smooth, creamy batter. Turn into the prepared tin and bake on the centre shelf for about 20–22 minutes. (A finger pressed on to the sponge will spring back when the cake is done.) Leave in the tin for 3 minutes then turn out on to a wire rack. Peel off the parchment and leave to grow cold. Cut in half and sandwich the two halves together with jam. Dust the top with icing sugar. Eat freshly baked or within 3 days of making. Store in an airtight container, loosely wrapped in food film or greaseproof.

Notes. See chapter 12 for how to dress it up for a celebration. For a larger sponge, double the ingredients and use 2 tins.

Victoria sponge (makes 6 slices) ***
A light, soft, golden sponge – always popular. The binders are pectin in the jam and eggs.

5 oz (140g) RG77 gluten-free flour blend (see chapter 3)
1½ level teaspoons gluten-free baking powder
4 oz (100g) polyunsaturated soft margarine
2 medium eggs, beaten
3oz (75g) jam-sugar with pectin
about 10 drops vanilla flavouring
rice flour for dusting

Method: Cut baking parchment to fit 2 round sponge tins, 6in (15cm). Grease the tins around the edges and flour with rice flour. Put in the parchment bases. Preheat oven at Gas 4/190° C/375° F. Put the flour and baking powder into a bowl and mix well. Add the margarine, eggs, sugar and flavouring. Mix/beat to a soft cream and divide between the two tins. Bake on a shelf above centre of the oven for about 25 minutes. (When a finger is pressed lightly into the top, the sponge will spring back if it is done.) Leave in the tin for 2 minutes to allow the edge to shrink a little. Go round the edge with a knife then turn out carefully on to a wire rack. Peel off the baking parchment and leave to cool. When cold, sandwich the two together with jam and dust the top with icing sugar or ice with white water icing. Expect a slightly crazed top but this does not affect texture or flavour. and it is part of its gluten-free character. See chapter 12 for Gateaux.

Victoria sponge II *** – Make as for Victoria sponge above but instead of jam-sugar with pectin use caster sugar. Add 4 pinches Xantham gum to the flour with the baking powder.

Fruit Cake – basic mix for a light, 1lb (500g) cake ***
A small cake baked in a loaf tin which will give 8 or 9 slices. Keeps well if made with dried fruit but must be eaten within 2 days if fresh fruit is used. A treat for elevenses, tea, a snack or in a lunchbox. Serve the fresh fruit cake as a dessert.

    1 level teaspoon gluten-free baking powder
    4 oz (100g) RG77 gluten-free flour blend
    ¼ level teaspoon Xanthan gum
    2 oz (50g) caster sugar
    2 oz (50g) polyunsaturated soft margarine
    2 medium eggs, beaten

finely grated rind of ½ lemon
4 oz (100g) fruit – see list below
granulated sugar for finishing

Method: Preheat oven at Gas 5/190° C/375° F. Line a small loaf tin with baking parchment. (Use a ½ lb/250g or a 1lb/500g size). Put the baking powder, flour, and Xanthan gum into a bowl and mix well. In a second bowl beat the sugar and margarine to a cream then add the flour, eggs and rind. Mix then beat to a smooth, creamy batter. Stir in the fruit of your choice from the list that follows. Turn into the prepared loaf tin and sprinkle the top with a little granulated sugar. Bake above centre shelf for about 25 minutes or until a skewer will come out clean. Turn out of the tin on to a wire rack to cool. When cold, wrap dried fruit cake in food film and store in an airtight tin or for a fresh fruit cake store wrapped in the fridge.

Dried fruit: 4 oz (100g) of any **one** of the following dried fruits – raisins, currants, sultanas, dried apricots (chopped), dried bluberries, dried cranberries.

Mixed dried fruit: 1 oz (25g) each of raisins, currants, sultanas, and chopped dried apricots plus finely grated rind of 1 orange.

Fresh fruit: use 4 oz (100g) ripe, sweet fruit
Pineapple – cut into small chunks, omit lemon peel; add
     about 8 drops vanilla flavouring.
Cherry – use stoned cherries cut into 4.
Peach – chopped small; add 5 drops vanilla flavouring
Plum – use destoned plums, chopped small.

Basic plain cake (makes 1 small loaf) ***
A light cake that can be flavoured. You will need a small loaf
tin 8 oz (250g) or an old fashioned 1lb (½ kilo) tin. (Double
the recipe for a larger tin and bake for a little longer.)

1 level teaspoon gluten-free baking powder
¼ level teaspoon Xanthan gum
2 oz (50g) polyunsaturated soft margarine
2 oz (50g) caster sugar
1 medium egg
4 oz (100g) RG77 gluten-free flour blend (see chapter 3)
1 tablespoon milk
flavouring of your choice – see list that follows
more RG77 flour for flouring tin

Method: Preheat oven at Gas 5/190° C/375° F. Grease and
flour the loaf tin. Put the first 7 ingredients into a bowl and
mix/beat to a smooth batter. Mix in the flavouring of your
choice. Turn into the prepared tin and bake above centre shelf
for about 20 minutes, then lower the heat to Gas 4/180°C/
375°F and bake for another 20 minutes until well risen. Test
with a skewer to see if it is done. If it comes out clean, it is.
Let the cake cool in the tin for 5 minutes then turn out on to
a wire rack to grow cold. Wrap in food film and store in an
airtight container. Use within 5 days.
    Flavourings – choose one from this list

Vanilla – add about 10 drops of vanilla flavouring.
Ginger – add 2 level teaspoons ground ginger and 1
    teaspoon golden syrup. (Warm the spoon.)
Chocolate – add 2 heaped teaspoons cocoa, 6 drops vanilla
    flavouring and 1 teaspoon golden syrup. (Warm the
    spoon.)
Spice – add 1 slightly heaped teaspoon mixed spice.

Orange – add the finely grated rind of 1 orange.

Lemon – add the finely grated rind of 1 lemon.

Seed – add 1 teaspoon caraway seeds and 1 teaspoon golden syrup. (Warm the spoon.)

Coffee – add 1 heaped teaspoon instant coffee (dissolved in the milk) and 1 teaspoon golden syrup. (Warm the spoon.)

Apple cake (makes 6 slices) ***

Sometimes there is a need for a cake that will please all the family and friends, not just the gluten-free dieter. This one is ideal and it can be served for tea or for a pudding with custard.

4 oz (100g) RG77 gluten-free flour blend (see chapter 3)

1 level teaspoon gluten-free baking powder

3 oz (75g) polyunsaturated soft margarine

2 oz (50g) jam-sugar with pectin

1 medium egg, beaten

6 oz (150g) peeled and cored cooking apple finely grated rind of ½ a lemon

Method: Preheat oven at Gas 4/180° C/350 °/F. Cut the apple into small dice or grate coarsely. Line the base of a sponge tin with baking parchment. Put the flour into a bowl, mix in the baking powder and rub in the margarine until it resembles crumbs. Mix in the sugar and lemon rind, then the egg. Lastly, stir in the apple. Turn into the prepared tin and bake on the top shelf for about 35 minutes. When baked turn out on to a wire rack to cool. Dust the top with icing sugar when cold. Eat within 2 days. Makes a moist cake. Keep wrapped in food film in the fridge. The fruit can be varied. Instead of apple use one of the following: fresh rhubarb using tender stalks, ripe plums, fresh peaches or nectarines, all cut into small pieces.

Lemon yoghurt cake (makes 6-8 slices) ***

A light, dainty show-off cake for elevenses or tea. Can also be served with fruit salad as a dessert cake or made into a lemon drizzle cake (see chapter 12).

> 2 oz (50g) polyunsaturated soft margarine
> 3 oz (75g) caster sugar
> 1 medium egg, beaten
> 1 level teaspoon gluten-free baking powder
> 5 oz (140g) RG77 gluten-free flour blend (see chapter 3)
> 4 oz (100g) set, unflavoured yoghurt
> finely grated rind of ½ a lemon
> 1½ tablespoons fresh lemon juice
> 1 oz (25g) ground almonds

Method: Preheat oven at Gas 4/180°C/350°F. Grease a small loaf tin size 3½ x 6½ inches (9 x 16 cm) with margarine. Put the margarine and sugar into a bowl and mix/beat to a cream. Add the egg, baking powder and flour and mix/beat to make a creamy batter. Carefully stir in the yoghurt, juice and rind (don't beat). Spoon into the prepared tin and bake on a shelf above centre for 45 minutes. Test with a skewer. If it comes out clean, the cake is baked. Leave to cool in the tin for 5 minutes then turn out on to a wire rack to cool. When cold, wrap in food film and store in an airtight container.

Rock buns (makes 5) cookies ***

Rugged and rustic looking buns meant to represent rocks, so no two are exactly alike. Very easy and quick to make. A good traveller, ideal for the lunchbox, school satchel or handbag.

Use for elevenses, tea or a snack. Make double the recipe and serve to the whole family.

2½ oz (75g) RG77 gluten-free flour blend (see chapter 3)
4 pinches Xanthan gum
1 level teaspoon ground almonds
1¼ oz (30g) polyunsaturated soft margarine
¾ oz (20g) caster sugar
½ medium beaten egg
finely grated rind of ¼ of a lemon
2 oz (50g) dried fruit from the list below
granulated or demerara sugar for finishing
rice flour for flouring etc.

Method: Line a baking tray with baking parchment. Put the RG77 flour into a bowl with the Xanthan gum and ground almonds. Mix well to combine. Add the margarine and rub in with the fingertips until the mixture resembles crumbs. Stir in the sugar. Add the egg and mix with a metal spoon to make a sticky dough. Put in the rind and dried fruit of your choice (see below). Mix into one sticky lump. Divide into 5 rough pieces and put on the prepared baking sheet with a teaspoon, leaving space around each one. Leave them rugged and sprinkle tops with sugar. Bake in a preheated oven at Gas 5/190 °C/375° F on the top shelf for about 15 minutes or until golden. (Do not let them brown or they will be too dry.) Take off the baking sheet and leave to cool on a wire rack. When cold, wrap each one in food film and store in an airtight container. Eat within 3 days.

Dried fruit: Use just one kind – currants, raisins, sultanas, chopped dried apricots, chopped destoned prunes, chopped dried blueberries. For a mixture, use what you have in the cupboard to make a weight of 2 oz (50g). Do not use glacé cherries or candied peel unless you are sure they are gluten-free.

Dried fruit and nut rock buns ***

Make as for rock buns but use 1 oz (25g) each of dried fruit and nuts. Chop nuts coarsely. Almonds, walnuts, hazelnuts, pecan are suitable, or a mixture – whatever is in your cupboard.

Cookies (makes 6) ***

A humble kind of cookie with pectin as the main binder. Easy to make and with 15 variations for fruit and flavour.

½ level teaspoon baking powder
3 oz (90g) RG77 gluten-free flour blend (see chapter 3)
spices of your choice (see list below)
1½ oz (40g) polyunsaturated soft margarine
1 oz (25g) jam-sugar with pectin (see chapter 2 for details)
2½ oz (75g) fresh or dried fruit of your choice (see list
    below)
finely grated rind ½ lemon
½ medium beaten egg
granulated sugar for finishing

Method: Line a baking tray with baking parchment. Grease with margarine. In a bowl mix the baking powder, flour and spices of your choice. Rub in the margarine until mixture resembles large breadcrumbs. Sprinkle in the jam-sugar, fruit and rind. Mix. Stir in the egg using a knife to make a stiff mixture. Make 6 heaps on the prepared baking tray, leaving space around each one for them to spread. Sprinkle tops with sugar and bake above centre shelf in preheated oven at Gas 5/180°C/375°F for about 15 minutes. When baked they will be pale in colour. Cool on a wire rack. When cold, wrap individually in food film and store in an airtight container. Eat within 2 days if fresh fruit is used and 5 days if dried fruit is used.

Note: Avoid baking them until they have browned as this will dry them out.

For the dried/fresh fruit and spices choose from the list below.

- Add 1 oz (25g) chopped, stoned dates and 1½ oz (40g) finely chopped eating apple
- Omit lemon rind. Add 2½ oz (75g) chopped fresh pear and 1 teaspoon cocoa.
- Add 2½ oz (75g) chopped dried apricots and 1 teaspoon cinnamon
- Add 2½ oz (75g) chopped, pitted prunes
- Omit lemon rind. Add 1 level teaspoon instant coffee dissolved in 1 teaspoon hot water and 2½ oz (65g) chopped walnuts
- Omit lemon rind. Add 6 drops vanilla flavouring and 2½ oz (75g) fresh pineapple cut into small cubes
- Add 1 oz (25g) fresh or defrosted blackcurrants and 1½ oz (40g) and 1½ oz (40g) finely chopped eating apple
- Add 1 oz (25g) fresh blackberries, chopped and 1½ oz (40g) finely chopped eating apple
- Add 2½ oz (75g) chopped, stoned dates and ½ level teaspoon ground ginger
- Add 1 oz (25g) each currants, raisins and sultanas
- Add 4 good pinches ground cloves and 2½ oz (65g) finely chopped eating apple
- Add 2½ oz (65g) defrosted berry mix
- Add 2½ oz (65g) dried blueberries
- Omit lemon rind. Add 1 slightly heaped teaspoon cocoa,

6 drops vanilla flavouring and 2½ oz (75g) stoned fresh black cherries, chopped
• Omit lemon rind. Add 6 drops vanilla flavouring, 1 slightly heaped teaspoon cocoa and 2 oz (50g) chopped hazelnuts

Note: Do not use glacé cherries or candied peel unless you are sure they are gluten-free. See chapter 3 for more information.

Hot cross buns – makes 5 (with yeast) ***
Semi-sweet, spicy, fruity Easter buns with a traditional cross and shiny top.

4½ oz (125g) RG77 gluten-free flour blend (see chapter 3)
1 heaped teaspoon ground almonds
½ level teaspoon gluten-free baking powder
¼ level teaspoon Xanthan gum
1 pinch salt
1 oz (25g) caster sugar
¼ level teaspoon cinnamon
1 level teaspoon mixed spice
finely grated rind of ½ a lemon
1 teaspoon gluten-free fast action instant yeast
1½ (40g) polyunsaturated soft margarine
1½ medium beaten eggs
1 oz 25g sultanas
1 oz (25g) currants
2 dried apricots cut into tiny cubes
more RG77 flour for kneading etc.
jelly from apricot jam for glazing

Method: Put the first ten ingredients into a bowl and mix well. Add the margarine and rub in until the mixture resembles crumbs. Add the egg and mix to a soft dough. Work in the fruit. Knead lightly for a minute, using more of the flour then divide into 5 and shape into buns. Place on a greased baking tray and make crosses on the top of each one (not too deep) with a sharp knife. Cover loosely with food film and a clean tea towel. Leave to rise in a warm place.

When doubled in size and the crosses have opened up, bake on the centre shelf of a preheated oven at Gas 5/190°C/375°F for about 12 – 15 minutes until golden. (Don't let them brown as they will be overbaked.) Put on to a wire rack and brush with the apricot jelly. Eat while still warm, split and buttered. Wrap cold buns in food film and use toasted the following day. They will toast quickly so need a low setting on the toaster.

Hot cross buns (makes 6) sponge type ***
If you don't want the trouble of making yeasted buns, make the sponge type. They are suitable for eating still warm but not for toasting. All the flavours of hot cross buns and the crosses too but gluten-free and different.

2½ oz (75g) RG77 gluten-free flour blend
1 oz (25g) caster sugar
2 oz (50g) polyunsaturated soft margarine
1 medium egg
2 pinches Xanthan gum
1 heaped teaspoon ground almonds
½ oz (15g) each of currants and sultanas
2 dried apricots cut into small cubes
finely grated rind of ¼ of a lemon
2 good pinches cinnamon
½ level teaspoon mixed spice
toasted flaked almonds for the crosses
apricot jam for glazing

Method: Preheat the oven at Gas 5/190°C/375°F. Line patty tins with 6 cake papers. Mix the first 6 ingredients in a bowl. Beat to a cream. Stir in the fruit, rind and spices. Divide between the paper cases. Make a cross on top of each one with flaked almonds. Bake on the top shelf for about 15-20 minutes, until well risen and golden. Transfer to a wire rack. Brush the tops with the jelly from apricot jam to make them shine. Serve still warm from the oven if you can.

BISCUITS

These began centuries ago as a form of dried bread, made from wheat and water, that could be taken on sea voyages and would make wheat keep for months. (The Great Fire of London in1666 started in a bakery making bulk biscuits for the navy. In the aftermath of the fire, when there was no bread to be had, the king ordered biscuits to be distributed to victims of the fire.) Nowadays biscuits are made with a lot of fat and a lot of sugar, except for crispbreads and semi-sweet versions.

Biscuits (makes about 12) crisp and flavoured (see list below)
***

pinch of salt
4 oz RG77 gluten-free flour blend (see chapter 3)
¼ teaspoon gluten-free baking powder
¼ teaspoon Xanthan gum
1 oz (25g) caster sugar
flavouring from the list below
1 oz (25g) polyunsaturated soft margarine
½ a beaten medium egg
1 tablespoon cold water
more of the RG77 flour for rolling out
caster sugar for finishing

Method: Preheat oven at Gas 6/200°C/400°F. Put the salt, flour, baking powder, Xanthan gum, sugar and flavouring into a bowl. Mix well and rub in the margarine until the mixture resembles breadcrumbs. Add the egg and water. Mix by hand and bring it together to make 1 ball of dough. (Don't be tempted to add more water, just keep going – it will take about a minute.) Dust the worktop with a little of the flour. Knead lightly for a few seconds until smooth. Roll out using more flour. Use a biscuit cutter or a tumbler to make round shapes. Place on an ungreased baking sheet and prick with a fork. Bake on the top shelf for 10 minutes, then turn the biscuits over and bake for another 5 minutes until they begin to turn brown around the edges. Put on to a wire rack to cool and sprinkle lightly with caster sugar. When cold, wrap individually in food film and store in an airtight container.

Flavourings:

- ½ level teaspoon mixed spice
- ½ teaspoon ground cinnamon
- finely grated rind of ¼ of a lemon or orange
- ½ level teaspoon ground ginger
- about 6 drops vanilla flavouring.

- For chocolate use just 3½ oz of the RG77 flour and 1 heaped teaspoon cocoa with a few drops of vanilla flavouring.

Moon biscuits (makes 16) show-off biscuits for the family and guests. ***
Strangely textured, unusual and very moreish.

5 oz (125g) RG77 gluten-free flour blend (see chapter 3)
2 level tablespoons ground almonds

¼ teaspoon Xanthan gum
2 oz (50g) polyunsaturated soft margarine
2 oz (50g) caster sugar
finely grated rind of ½ an orange
about 10 drops vanilla flavouring
1 medium egg, beaten
2 oz (50g) gluten-free cooking chocolate chips
caster sugar for finishing
more RG77gluten-free flour for kneading etc.

Method: Preheat oven at Gas 6/200°C/400°F. Line 2 baking trays with baking parchment. Put the flour, ground almonds and Xanthan gum into a bowl and mix well to distribute evenly. Add the margarine and rub in with the fingertips until the mixture resembles crumbs. Sprinkle in the sugar, rind and vanilla flavouring. Mix then add the egg to make a sticky dough, using a metal spoon. Work in the chocolate chips by hand and using more of the flour, shape into 2 sausages. Cut off 8 thick slices from both and roll each slice into a ball. Flatten with the palms and fingers to make round biscuit shapes. Try to make them all the same size. Place on the prepared baking trays and bake on the top shelf for about 15 minutes. They should be pale but just starting to brown around the edges. (You may need to turn the trays in the oven to get even baking after the first 10 minutes.) Leave to cool and crisp on a wire rack. Serve with tea or coffee as a treat.

Note: If the baking has begun to melt the chocolate chips, don't worry, they will set again as the biscuits cool down – this is what gives the biscuits their characteristic appearance. Best eaten on the day of baking but individually wrapped in food film they will stay crisp for a few days

Dessert biscuits (makes about 12) ***
Quickly baked, light, crisp and dainty biscuits to serve with ice cream, sorbets, fruit salad etc.

2 oz (50g) RG77 gluten-free flour blend (see chapter 3)
1 pinch gluten-free baking powder
1 pinch Xanthan gum
1 oz (25g) polyunsaturated soft margarine
1 oz (25g) caster sugar
white of 1 medium egg, lightly beaten
about 6 drops vanilla flavouring

Method: Preheat oven at Gas 7/220° C/425° F. Grease 2 baking sheets. Put the flour into a basin with the baking powder and Xanthan gum. Mix well to distribute. Use a mixing bowl to cream the margarine and sugar. Add the egg white and flour mixture. Mix/beat to a smooth cream, using a metal tablespoon. Put in the vanilla flavouring and mix again. Use a teaspoon to put spoonfuls on to the prepared baking sheets, leaving space around each one. Spread them out thinly using the back of the teaspoon. Keep them more or less the same size and shape for even baking – round, oblong or oval. Bake on the top shelf of the oven for about 10 minutes or until pale cream with golden brown edges. Loosen with a knife and transfer to a wire rack to grow cold and crisp. Store individually wrapped in food film, in an airtight container. Eat within a week.

Note: You will need to keep a close eye on these as they bake so quickly. Turn the trays round after 7 minutes to bake them evenly brown round the edges.

Macaroons (makes 5) ****

Either make these on rice paper (check label) or baking parchment. You can eat the former but not the latter. They don't have to be the traditional almond – walnuts, hazelnuts, pistachios, pecan or a mixture might be more interesting. They should be ground in a coffee grinder or mini food processor. (Commercial mixed nuts are usually heavy on peanuts and are perhaps best avoided.)

1 egg white
small pinch salt
1 oz (25g) caster sugar
½ oz (15g) rice flour
1½ oz (40g) plain, ground nuts
pieces of nut for decoration

Method: Preheat oven at Gas 2/150° C/300° F. Line a baking tray with rice paper or baking parchment. Whisk the egg white with a hand beater until stiff. Add half the sugar and whisk again. Put in the remaining sugar and whisk again. Use a metal spoon to *fold* in the rice flour and the nuts. Make 5 heaps on the prepared baking sheet, leaving space around each one for them to spread. Spread out with the back of the spoon and put a piece of appropriate nut in the centre. Bake for about 30 minutes above centre shelf. When dark gold transfer to a wire rack to cool. When cold, if you have used rice paper, trim off excess with kitchen scissors otherwise peel off baking parchment. Store in an airtight container and eat within 2 weeks. Wrap individually in food film.

Note: The macaroons can be flavoured. If using almonds add 3 drops of almond flavouring. For walnuts add 3 pinches instant coffee. A level teaspoon of cocoa goes well with hazelnuts.

Ratafias ****

Make the macaroon recipe with almonds and 3 drops almond flavouring but make into 20 very small macaroons and bake for less time – about 15 minutes. Use for decorating trifles, or just as little biscuits.

Gingersnaps (makes 10) crisp, crunchy traditional biscuits **

    1 oz (25g) polyunsaturated margarine
    1 oz (25g) soft brown sugar
    1 level tablespoon golden syrup (warm the spoon)
    3 oz (75g) RG77 gluten-free flour blend (see chapter 3)
    ¼ level teaspoon bicarbonate of soda
    pinch salt
    2 pinches Xanthan gum
    ¼ level teaspoon ground ginger

Method: Preheat oven at Gas 4/180°C/350°F. Grease a baking sheet. Put the margarine, sugar and syrup into a small saucepan. Set over a gentle heat and stir until melted and blended. Put aside to cool a little. Put the flour, bicarbonate of soda, salt, Xanthan gum and ginger into a bowl. Mix well and add the mixture from the pan. Mix to a soft dough. Use 2 tea-spoons to put 10 neat mounds of the dough on to the prepared baking sheet, leaving enough space around each one for spreading. Put into the oven on the top shelf and bake for about 15 minutes. They will form into neat, round biscuits. Cool on the baking sheet for 2 minutes then loosen with a

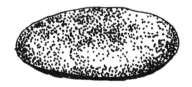

palette knife and transfer to a wire rack to cool and grow crisp and crunchy. When cold, wrap individually in food film and store in an airtight container. Eat within 4 days.

Tart du Jour (4-6 servings) ***

A very attractive tart to serve as a snack, dessert or tea.

Make the shortcrust pastry from chapter 3. Roll out on a sheet of baking parchment and transfer on to a baking sheet. Trim with a sharp knife to make a square or oblong shape. Pinch up the edge all round between thumb and forefinger. Bake in a preheated oven at Gas 7/220° C/425° F for about 12 – 15 minutes and before it begins to brown. Put on to a wire rack to cool and when cold, put on to a serving plate. Make some thick custard and allow to cool a little. Spread thickly over the pastry. Cover with ripe, fresh fruit in lines, overlapping where necessary – peeled, sliced kiwi fruit, halved strawberries, blueberries, raspberries, sliced fresh peaches, canned apricot halves, sliced or canned sliced peaches (both drained). Heat 2 tablespoons redcurrant jelly and brush over the fruit to glaze. Leave to set for 30 minutes. Serve in slices on its own. Eat freshly made.

Note: The jelly part of apricot jam can be used instead of the redcurrant jelly.

To make the custard use about half the amount of milk you would normally use. See chapter 8.

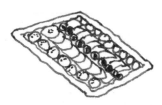

Tartlets (makes 6) ***

See chapter 3 for shortcrust pastry. Bake 6 little cases. (The longer this pastry is baked the more it will dry out, so it should be cream in colour not browned.) When cold use for the following:

Jam tarts – put a generous teaspoon of jam into each one. **

Strawberry tartlets – see chapter 12.

Treacle tarts – put a generous teaspoon golden syrup into each one and a teaspoon crushed gluten-free cornflakes. *

Little pies (makes 4) **

Apple pies – bake the pastry cases and lids. When still warm fill the cases with sweetened stewed apple and put on the lids. Sprinkle the tops with caster sugar. ***

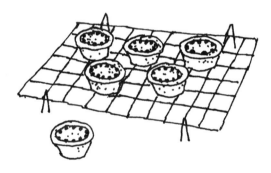

Mince pies – make the pastry cases, before baking fill each one with a generous teaspoon of gluten-free home-made mincemeat. Put on the lids and bake for about 10 minutes. Cool on a wire rack. When cold, dust with icing sugar. See chapter 14 for gluten-free recipe for sweet mincemeat. **

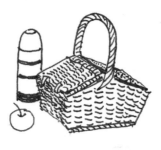

CHAPTER 11

Packed Meals and Picnics

To most people this kind of food means sandwiches with wheat bread, a packet of crisps and a piece of fruit (perhaps), a bun or pastry or piece of cake, a bar of chocolate and/or biscuits. Oh dear!

Packed meals/picnics are a godsend to the gluten-free dieter who is not able to always eat out safely, the traveller and he schoolchild. It is always a food eaten away from home and has particular requirements. It should be sustaining, a delight to eat, nutritious and often be suitable to eat with the fingers, sometimes off a picnic plate but more often out of a container or bag. It should also be food which will travel without spoiling. There should be a familiar bag, basket or container for all the food etc. Buy in ironmongers, or stores. For hot weather an insulated 'cool box' is invaluable, as is a vacuum flask, which can be used for both hot and cold drinks or just hot water to make a cup of tea or coffee.

Plastic bags, greaseproof paper, food film, plastic containers, screwtop plastic jars, kitchen paper, a plastic bottle for water, teaspoon, knife fork and spoon, plastic or enamel plate, bowls, a small screwtop container for dried milk and another for tea or coffee bags, tiny salt and pepper containers, a cup (there's usually one on the top of a flask). These are all you need although not all at once. As they have to be carried use ones as light as possible. Keep them scrupulously clean, washing them up after every use and putting them back into the bag/basket/container. Paper serviettes and hand wipes are always useful and so is a plastic bag in which to put fruit peelings, empty yoghurt pots, used tea bags etc. Make a list of the things you *might* possibly need to pack a meal and keep it in the kitchen so you can check it. There's nothing more disappointing than finding something has been left out when you are miles away from home.

It should read something like this:

tea/coffee bags, dried milk, flask of hot water, teaspoon, mug
savoury food, salad dressing, box of salad, gluten-free bread/rice/potatoes
flask of hot soup or a cold drink
fruit, fruit juice, yoghurt, cookie or piece of cake
paper serviettes, hand wipes, kitchen paper
plate, bowl, knife fork, spoon, teaspoon, fruit knife
freezer pack, cool box
bottle of water
salt and pepper

You shouldn't need *all* of these at any one time but it will help you to make sure everything is in for a particular packed lunch.

Things to bear in mind
Avoid too much stodgy, sugary or salty food. A packed meal should leave you feeling refreshed and comfortable, ready to face the rest of the day, not thirsty, too full up and tired.

Some foods are not good travellers. Pears are a good example as they bruise easily. Some soups do not improve with waiting in a flask for hours. Delicate bakery items will not withstand a journey and consequently disintegrate on the way.

- Stewed fruit can be taken in a small container.
- Salads can be packed in a box in an insulated container (if the weather is hot)but the dressing must be carried in a small jar ready to pour over when required, not before. If fruit to be peeled is not a good idea then fruit salad can be packed in a jar, ready to eat with a spoon. ****
- Fruit yoghurt can be made at home with unflavoured yoghurt and a heaped tablespoon of finely chopped or pureed fruit stirred in with a *little* sugar to taste. Spoon into a jar and make sure you put in a teaspoon. ***
- Hard boiled egg, cold plain cooked meat or low-fat cheese, canned salmon, tuna (in oil and not sauce) and nuts all make a good high protein food. One of these should be part of the meal. Cut the meat into bite-sized pieces for convenience. They can all be put into sandwiches and rolls/baps or packed in a small container to eat with salad. Use gluten-free chutney with the cold meats and gluten-free light mayonnaise with the fish for the sandwiches. (See chapter 8). ****
- Freshly made gluten-free baps or rolls as well as bread will travel well, wrapped tightly in food film. They can be filled before being packed or filled just before eating if the filling is taken separately in a small container. ***
- Gluten-free bread is not essential if this is difficult, as you can use cold boiled rice and cold boiled potatoes with a little salad dressing and a teaspoon of finely chopped onion. Both are good with small boxes of salad vegetables. ***
- Gluten-free pasties are good travellers. Wrap in food

film after baking as soon as they are cold. (See chapter 3 for pastry and chapter 7 for pasties). If you can't wait for them to grow cold, wrap in greaseproof paper, not food film.
- See chapter 4 for muesli. This will travel dry and the milk can be put on just before eating. Slice up a banana to put on the top or use other fruit. ****

If the gluten-free dieter has to make an early start from home you can make the food in its containers the evening before and store in the fridge overnight. This is not as good as freshly made that morning but sometimes it is the only way to cope.

Picnics
These are slightly more complicated than just packed meals. The special gluten-free food needs to be kept separate. If it is a family/friends picnic it helps if some of the food can be eaten by everyone, such as fruit salad.

Prepare any gluten-free food which is just for the gluten-free dieter and no one else. Pack it first and keep it separate. If it is a teatime picnic make gluten-free buns for *everyone* – see chapter 10, or strawberry tarts. A picnic is a 'together' thing so the gluten-free dieter should be made to feel part of it and not a nuisance by requiring different food from everyone else. Eating the same food is part of that. Make the picnic a pleasurable event with as much food that *everyone* can enjoy as is possible.

Sandwich fillings etc.
See chapter 8 for the light mayonnaise recipe.

- grated low-fat cheddar cheese and gluten-free chutney or tomato slices or cooked beetroot, sliced

- lettuce, hard boiled egg and tomato slices with gluten-free light mayonnaise ****
- hard boiled egg slices with cress or watercress, chopped, and gluten-free light mayonnaise ****
- hard boiled egged mashed with a little gluten-free light mayonnaise and 3 or 4 pinches medium curry powder ****
- pâté from chapter 5
- mashed cottage cheese and chopped stoned dates, 1 per sandwich ****
- mashed cottage cheese and 1 finely chopped walnut per sandwich ****
- drained, canned sardines in oil mashed with a squeeze of fresh lemon juice and a little gluten-free light mayonnaise ****
- drained, canned tuna in oil, mashed with a little gluten-free light mayonnaise ****
- drained canned salmon, mashed with a squeeze of lemon juice and thin slices of cucumber ****
- cold roast meat slices – beef, pork, chicken, ham (without breadcrumb coating) etc. and gluten-free corned beef with gluten-free chutney or chopped tomato and shredded lettuce or watercress sprigs. ****

To keep sandwiches daisy fresh, put into a plastic bag and seal. Wrap the bag in 2 sheets of kitchen paper dipped in cold water and gently wrung out. Put into another slightly larger bag. Keep closed with a clothes-peg until required.

Other foods to take are gluten-free pasties, (see chapter 7), a small can of gluten-free baked beans (***) and a can-opener/spoon, cold omelet with a salad. (****) In summer use the vacuum flask for iced cold drinks of fruit juice or water and in winter for hot soup or hot water to make a coffee or tea.

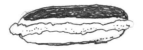

CHAPTER 12

Celebrations and Entertaining

Some of the recipes in this chapter can be regarded as posh junkfood. They are not food for everyday but once in a while they can be eaten as a treat, not just by the gluten-free dieter but *everyone* at the celebration.

Parties for children, grownups, special occasions, tea parties, dinner parties, suppers, buffets – all times to make a special effort and times to remember. Some of the recipes for these are in previous chapters but the very special ones are in this one. Used too often, they will no longer be a treat, so use sparingly and make them even more memorable.

The big show-off desserts should be exciting such as Pavlova and Gateau. Some can be retro like trifle and baked Alaska and others can be more up to date. Take trouble to present them well – this is part of the magic and the memories.

Suggested menus are at the end of the chapter and they are all gluten-free.

Pavlova – serves 8 **

meringue:
4 egg whites
8 oz (250g) caster sugar
1 tablespoon cornflour
2 teaspoons wine vinegar
few drops vanilla flavouring
filling:
10 fluid oz (275ml) whipping cream
3 pinches caster sugar
fresh fruit of your choice (see below)

Method: Line a baking sheet with baking parchment. Preheat oven at Gas 2/150°C/300°F. Put the egg whites into a bowl and whisk until stiff. Begin to add the sugar, a tablespoon at a time, whisking after each addition. When the meringue is very stiff, whisk in the cornflour, vinegar and vanilla flavouring. Make a pile of the meringue on the baking parchment. Use a palette knife to spread it out into a circle about 9 inches (23cm) across. Slightly hollow out the centre and bake below the centre shelf for about 1½ hours. (This is more of a drying out process than baking.) Leave to cool. When cold, remove the paper and place on a serving dish. Whip the cream with the sugar until stiff. Fold in some of the fruit. Pile into the centre hollow of the meringue and decorate with the remaining fruit. Serve with a knife and a cake slice.

Fruit: choose a mixture or all one kind of fruit. Classic favourite is fresh strawberries. Raspberries are also very showy but you can also use passion fruit and small cubes of fresh pineapple. Fruit should be ripe, fresh and sweet.

Sherry trifle (serves 6) **
Make the vanilla flavoured fairy cakes from chapter 10.

strawberry jam
3 tablespoons sherry
1 small tin of peach slices or apricot halves, drained
1 pint (600ml) thick custard (see chapter 9)
¼ pint (150ml) whipping cream
finishing:
ratafias (see recipe in chapter !0)
toasted almond flakes
halved red seedless grapes – about 5 or 6

Method: Use 3 of the fairy cakes. Cut in half and sandwich with jam. Break into pieces and put into the bottom of a glass bowl. Spoon over the sherry and top with the fruit, cut into pieces. Cover with custard and leave to grow cold. Whip the cream and spread over the cold custard. Decorate the top with grape halves round the edge, alternating with the little ratafias. Sprinkle the nuts in the centre.

Note: Most commercial ratafias contain wheat and are not gluten-free. (See chapter 10 for recipe.) For a non-alcoholic version use pineapple juice instead of sherry.

Celebration cake (makes a 6in (15 cm) round cake) **
A traditional cake for covering in marzipan and icing. For Christmas, birthdays and weddings etc. Because the gluten-free flour is such a small part of the recipe, the resulting cake is indistinguishable from an ordinary rich fruit cake of this kind. If you have to bake one for an important celebration, I suggest you have a practice with this small version. (For a larger cake double the amounts and use an 8 in (20.5 cm) tin.) It will take 3 hours or more to bake so pick a day when you don't need your oven for that amount of time.

2 fluid oz (50ml) sherry
4 oz (100g) polyunsaturated margarine
4½ oz (120g) soft brown sugar
1 tablespoon black treacle (warm the spoon)
6 oz (170g) sultanas
5 oz (140g) currants
5 oz (140g) raisins
3 oz (75g) dried apricots, cut into small cubes
juice and finely grated rind of ½ an orange
juice and finely grated rind of ½ a lemon
2 oz(50g) ground almonds
2 oz(50g) shelled almonds, chopped coarsely
5½ oz (155g) RG77 gluten-free flour blend
½ teaspoon mixed spice
¼ teaspoon nutmeg
1 pinch ground ginger
2 large eggs, beaten
¼ teaspoon almond flavouring
milk or apple juice to mix, if required

Method: Place a large saucepan on the hob. Put in the sherry, margarine, sugar, treacle, dried fruit, citrus rinds and juice. Gently melt the margarine and bring to the boil while you stir. Lower heat and simmer for 10 minutes, stirring from tme to time. Turn into a large mixing bowl and leave to cool for an hour. Prepare the tin. Grease and line with baking parchment, allowing 2in (5cm) extra height above the level of the tin. In a large basin, mix the ground and chopped almonds with the spices and flour. Stir the eggs and almond flavouring into the cooled fruit mixture. Add the flour and stir well. Turn into the prepared tin and flatten the top with the back of a metal spoon. Bake for an hour at Gas 2/150°C/300°F on the centre shelf, then turn down the heat to Gas 1/150°C/275°F. and cover the top loosely with greaseproof paper. Continue baking for another 1¾ hours – 2 hours. Test with a skewer straight down into the middle to see if it is done. If the skewer comes out clean, it is ready to come out of the oven. If not, continue baking. When baked, put on to a wire rack and leave to cool in the tin. (This will take several hours.) When cold, take out of the tin and wrap in a double layer of greaseproof paper. Put into an airtight container to mature. After 2 days, feed the cake. Unwrap and prick the top of the cake with a fork in several places to make little holes. Dribble a spoonful of brandy or sherry over it. It will run into the holes and disappear. The cake should be ready in 10 days but will keep much longer, wrapped and in an airtight container. Feed the cake again after a week, if you wish. A few days before you want to ice it, level off the top with a breadknife. Use a pastry brush to paint all over with apricot jam. This is to hold the marzipan. Roll out the marzipan (see following recipe) using icing sugar. Cover the cake and leave to harden for 1 or 2 days. Put on to a cake board and cover with royal icing. Any decorations should be gluten-free.

Note: If you don't want to cover the whole cake with marzipan and icing, just cover the top and use a cake frill for the sides. *Do not fix the frill on with pins.*

Marzipan/almond paste (makes 11 oz (325g)) enough for all over the celebration cake above. **
Commercial almond paste may not be gluten-free, is usually coloured bright yellow and amazingly smooth. The homemade variety is a natural beige colour and not quite so smooth but is far superior to the commercial kind. It is very easy to make.

3 oz (75g) caster sugar
2 oz (75g) icing sugar
6oz (175g) ground almonds
1 egg yolk

about 2 drops almond flavouring
1 teaspoon fresh lemon juice
more icing sugar for kneading etc.

Method: Mix the 2 sugars with the ground almonds in a bowl. Use a cup to mix the egg yolk with the almond flavouring and lemon juice. Make a well in the sugar/almond mixture in the bowl. Spoon in the egg mixture and mix well with a metal spoon to make a sticky paste. Turn out on to the worktop sprinkled lightly with icing sugar and knead by hand for about 3 minutes. Store in the fridge wrapped in food film. Keeps well but is inclined to harden if kept too long. Use to cover rich fruit cakes such as Christmas and traditional birthday cakes.

Royal Icing *(makes enough for 2 coats or 'frosting' for a 6 in (15cm) cake, all over. (No stars)*
2 egg whites
1 lb (500g) icing sugar
1 teaspoon lemon juice

Method: Beat the egg whites with a fork until frothy. Gradually beat in half the icing sugar, using a wooden spoon. Beat in the remaining sugar with the lemon juice. Beat well until smooth and white. Cover the bowl with a clean damp tea towel and leave to stand for a few hours. Any air bubbles will rise to the surface and burst. Before using, beat again with a wooden spoon, but don't overbeat.

Profiteroles (makes 20 to serve 5) *

Choux pastry cases:
Make double the recipe for choux pastry in chapter 3

Chocolate sauce:
6 oz (175g) plain, gluten-free chocolate
¼ pint (150ml) water
1 teaspoon instant coffee powder
4 oz (100g) caster sugar

Filling:
1 tablespoon sifted icing sugar
3 drops vanilla flavouring
6 fluid oz (170 ml) whipping cream

Method: Chop the chocolate and put into a small pan with 2 tablespoons of the water and the coffee. Gently heat until melted then add the remaining water and sugar. Continue to heat gently until the sugar has dissolved. Simmer for 10 minutes and leave to cool. Make the filling. Whip the cream until thick and fold in the sugar and flavouring. Pipe or spoon a little into each profiterole. Pile on to a serving dish and pour over the chocolate sauce.

Strawberry tart (6 slices) **
Make the shortcrust pastry from chapter 3. Bake blind but don't overbake – it should be pale. When cold brush with melted redcurrant jelly or apricot jam. Arrange halved strawberries to cover and brush with more of the jam to make a glaze. Pipe whipped cream around the edge.

Crépes Suzette **
See chapter 9. The gluten-free pancakes can be made in advance and stacked on a plate until required. The sauce can be made ready to warm up. For a *spectacular* finish, which takes some courage, add 2 tablespoons of Grand Marnier and 2 tablespoons of brandy to the sauce left in the pan. Heat gently then set fire to it with a match. Take great care

and pour the flaming liquid over the folded crepes in a heated ovenproof dish. Serve immediately on warmed plates.

Note: Best to practice this one first! For adults only.

Tart du Jour
See chapter 9

Summerfruit dessert (6 servings) ***
This is a very light pudding.

Make the whisked sponge from chapter 10. Serve in wedges with a heaped tablespoon of defrosted summerfruits on top and a blob of whipped cream.

Exotic fruit salad ****
See chapter 9. There's always somebody who won't like the show-off dessert. This is a back-up, very colourful and refreshing. (Some people will have both.)

Meringue baskets (makes 8) *
A useful recipe as the meringues can be baked ahead and filled as required.

meringue:
4 egg whites
about 5 drops vanilla flavouring
9 oz (275g) icing sugar
filling:
¼ pint (150ml) whipping cream
about 4 oz (100g) fresh, ripe small strawberries
2 tablespoons redcurrant jelly (jam)

Method: Line a baking sheet with baking parchment. Draw 8 x 3in (7.5cm) circles on the parchment. Heat ⅓ of a pan of water on the hob. Whisk the egg whites until stiff. Whisk in the vanilla flavouring and then the icing sugar, a tablespoon at a time, whisking after every addition. When the water has boiled in the pan lower the heat to simmer and place the bowl over it. Whisk for 5 minutes until the meringue is really stiff. Pile the meringue into little heaps, guided by the circles and making a well in the centre of each one. Use the tines of a fork to swirl round each one. Bake in a preheated oven at Gas 2/150°C/300°F for up to 1 hour or more to dry out. Cool on a wire rack before removing the paper. To finish, spoon a little whipped cream into the bottom of each one. Arrange the strawberries on top. Warm the redcurrant jelly and use a pastry brush to glaze the strawberries. Eat on the day of making.

Note: An alternative way to shape the baskets is to use half the meringue to cover the circles and use the remaining meringue in a piping bag with a large fluted nozzle, to pipe circles around the edge of each base. After baking and growing cold the meringues can be stored in an airtight container for several days.

Fruit kebabs *****
Not everyone wants to eat rich foods at a celebration. These look wonderful and are actually healthy as well as gluten-free and refreshing. You will need wooden skewers or smooth metal skewers (not meat skewers), or even cocktail sticks if you want to make small ones. Wash all the fruit before preparing.

Cut up a fresh, ripe and sweet pineapple, take off the outside and take out the core. Cut into bite sized chunks. Medium sized ripe strawberries and larger raspberries, destoned cherries, seedless grapes. Peel small clementines and separate the segments. If you are short on fresh fruit, drain a can of apricot halves and cut in half. Thread a selection on to the skewers or cocktail sticks. On the long skewers use the same selection and the same order. For the cocktail sticks just put 2 or 3 on and vary them. Arrange on a white plate. Colours of the fruit will be brilliant.

Ice cream

Gluten-free ice cream can be bought from supermarket freezers if you know which brand is gluten-free. If you would rather make your own, here are two recipes, both easy. Mainly ice cream comprises fat, sugar and a little flavouring. In terms of junkfood it is the ultimate. Think of it as an occasional treat, not an everyday food.

Gluten-free vanilla ice cream (makes 8 or 9 servings) *
This is rather high in cholesterol and not the slightest bit healthy so serve sparingly and rarely.

    3 oz (75g) caster sugar
    2 eggs
    2 egg yolks
    ¾ pint (450 ml) single cream
    5 or 6 drops vanilla flavouring
    10 fluid oz (280 ml) double cream for whipping

Method: Put the sugar, eggs and egg yolks into a bowl and mix well. Pour the single cream into a small pan and heat gently up to (not over) boiling point. Stir the egg mixture while you pour in the hot cream. Stir really well. Strain it through a wire mesh sieve into a clean bowl and stir in the flavouring. Leave to cool. When it is cold, whip the double cream until stiff and fold into the cold mixture. Pour into a rigid container that has a lid and will withstand the freezer. Freeze for about an hour then take it out of the freezer, give it a good stir and put it back into the freezer. Before using put into the fridge for 20 minutes just to soften it a little. Serve on its own or with fruit and dessert biscuits from chapter 10. Use for Baked Alaska. Store in the freezer, named and dated.

Gluten-free Budget Vanilla Ice Cream *

Sugar is already in the condensed milk so no more needs to be added.

1 small can full cream condensed milk
¼ pint (150ml) cold water
½ pint (300ml) evaporated milk (from cans)
about 8 drops vanilla flavouring

Method: Mix the condensed milk with the water and leave in the fridge overnight to cool. Pour the evaporated milk into a bowl, add the flavouring and whip until thick. Fold (don't beat yet) into shallow freezer containers and freeze until thick. Turn out into a bowl and beat until smooth. Return to the containers and re-freeze. Use for Baked Alaska and for a treat with dessert wafers (see chapter 10).

(Commercial ice cream wafers are usually made with wheat flour and are not gluten-free.)

Baked Alaska 6-8 servings *

This is a novelty dessert which is hot on the outside and cold on the inside. It needs to be served immediately it comes out of the oven so is only suitable for a dinner party. Putting cold ice cream into a hot oven takes a bit of nerve. If there is a little hole or a gap in the meringue then the ice cream will start to melt and run out. When you put it together you need to work quickly. Best to have practice with this one. The ice cream, sponge and raw meringue can all be made ahead and the fruit put ready. Put it together just before you want to bake and serve it.

base:
gluten-free sponge from chapter 10
1 medium can peach slices, drained
gluten-free vanilla ice cream from chapter 12
meringue:
4 egg whites
8 oz (250g) caster sugar
½ teaspoon vanilla flavouring

Method: Make a whisked sponge from chapter 10 for the base, using a square 8 in (19cm) tin. When cold put into a shallow ovenproof dish. Make the meringue. Whisk the egg whites in a large bowl until stiff. Carry on whisking until they don't slide about, if you tilt the bowl. Add the sugar, one tablespoon at a time, whisking after every addition. Finally whisk in the flavouring. The meringue should be glossy and form soft peaks. Cover the sponge with drained, canned sliced peaches. Top with gluten-free vanilla ice cream about 1 in (2.5cm) thick. Working quickly, cover the ice cream and fruit with the meringue, completely enclosing them. Use the tines of a fork to pull the meringue into little peaks. Immediately put into a hot oven preheated at Gas 6/200° C/400 °F for 3 or 4 minutes until the peaks of meringue begin to brown. Serve immediately.

Gateau **
Bake 2 sponges from chapter 3 – Victoria sponge or quick golden sponge. When cold, sandwich sponges with whipped cream and chopped fresh fruit. Cover the top with whipped cream. Decorate with whole fruit – strawberries or raspberries, or drained, canned apricot halves round the edge. Sprinkle with toasted flaked almonds in the centre. Serve with a cake fork.

Note: Other fruit to use – peeled, ripe kiwi fruit, sliced, small cubes of sweet fresh pineapple, canned peach slices.

Black Forest Gateau **
Bake 2 chocolate sponges – see chapter 10. Spread bottom half with whipped cream. Top with destoned black cherries, chopped. Put on the second sponge. Cover top with more whipped cream and decorate with halved, destoned black cherries. Defrosted fruits of the forest or summerfruits will do just as well. Assemble at the last minute as the juice may run from the fruit.

Buttercream *
Make as much as you need at one time of this very rich filling and topping. This is enough for a sponge filling or topping for 6 cupcakes. Extreme junkfood!

2 oz (50g) butter
3 oz (75g) icing sugar
2 teaspoons single cream (optional)

Method: Put the icing sugar on to a plate and crush with the back of a metal spoon to get out the lumps. Cut the butter into small pieces on a saucer. Warm a basin and put in the butter and about half the icing sugar. Mix/beat to a cream. Gradually beat in the other half of the icing sugar, flavouring of your choice and the cream if using. It should be a firm but light cream for spreading, texturing. and piping. Choose one of the flavourings – vanilla is the most popular.
Flavourings: 5 drops vanilla flavouring/ finely grated rind of ¼ of a lemon or orange/ 1 teaspoon instant coffee dissolved in ½ teaspoon hot water/ ½ teaspoon cocoa.

Sponge with jam and buttercream filling *
Bake the Victoria sponge from chapter 10. Put one half, top side down on to a plate lined with a paper doily. Spread with vanilla buttercream. Spread the base of the second sponge

with raspberry jam. Turn upside down on to the buttercream. Dust the top sponge with icing sugar.

Nibbles have already been dealt with in chapter 4 – chapati crisps, cheese straws, snax, and toasted nuts.

- See also vegetable dips (*****) in chapter 5 to arrange on a large plate and chapter 8 for dipping sauces – curry mayonnaise and pink mayonnaise
- Wrap cubes of ripe melon in a small piece of parma ham and secure with a cocktail stick. Arrange on a plate. ****
- Skewer cooked king prawns on cocktail sticks and arrange on a plate around a bowl of pink mayonnaise. ***
- Buy plain gluten-free potato crisps in the supermarket. Check label.
- Buy plain (not stuffed) pitted olives, green or black, in brine. Drain and put into bowls with a container of cocktail sticks and a small bowl or plate for the used sticks. Use small cherry tomatoes in the same way. A bowl of black olives with cherry tomatoes looks stunning.

Canapés *** down to * depending on topping
Served at cocktail/drinks parties or before a dinner party or at a reception, these bite-sized and moreish nibbles need to look attractive with bright colours. Allow 6 canapes per person and not less than 3 different kinds.

Here are a few ideas. See chapter 3 for canapé bases made from dropscone batter. These can be made well in advance. You can also use squares of gluten-free bread, fried on one side in a little sunflower oil. (These are better than toast which has the habit of going soggy.) Buy a cream cheese which is just that – a cream cheese and not a cheese spread with additives which may include gluten. If you feel the cream cheese is too thick, thin down with a little cream but don't make it *too* soft. You may need to buy this from a cheese counter rather than the shelves, already packed. Snip chives and put ready in a small bowl. Do the same with parsley, chopping it finely. Have your cocktail sticks to hand. Get the plates ready so you can put the canapés on them as soon as they are made.

- Spread canapé bases with cream cheese and top with a prawn, or a small piece of smoked salmon and a few of drops of lemon juice with a sprinkle of snipped chives.
- Spread canapé bases with gluten-free pâté (see recipes). Top with a slice of tomato from a very small cherry tomato and sprinkle with finely chopped parsley.
- Make mini choux pastry buns (as for profiteroles but smaller), fill each one with ½ a teaspoon of gluten-free creamed horseradish sauce (check label) and a small piece of cold roast beef, folded.
- Make tiny sandwiches from gluten-free bread (see chapter 3) with the crusts cut off to spear on cocktail sticks. Instead of spreading the bread with butter or margarine, use gluten-free mayonnaise (see chapter 4 for this and sandwich fillings).
- Spread canapé bases with cream cheese, cover with smoked salmon and a couple of drops of of lemon juice. Top with a blob of caviar and a sprinkle of snipped chives. Arrange on a plate with a sprig of parsley or watercress in the centre. Allow plenty of time to make as these are they are fiddly, but well worth the effort.

Presentation for canapés
Lay them out in circles or lines on plates. Use sprigs of parsley or watercress to decorate. If you have a garden, in season,

use nasturtium flowers about 3 to a plate. These give a splash
of colour. (They are edible and gluten-free.)

Nougat (makes about ¾ lb (330g)) *

8 oz (250g) shelled almonds
4 oz (100g) granulated sugar
½ teaspoon finely grated lemon rind
small pinch ground cinnamon
small pinch nutmeg
4 tablespoons runny honey
1 egg white, beaten until stiff
gluten-free edible rice paper

Method: Toast the almonds in the oven preheated at Gas
6/200° C/400° F for 6 minutes. Cool then chop coarsely. Mix
with the sugar, rind and spices in a bowl. Spoon the honey
into a small saucepan and warm it gently over a low heat. Stir
in the nut mixture and heat until the sugar has dissolved. Boil
until the mixture turns golden. Draw off the heat and fold in
the egg white. Pour into a shallow tin lined with rice paper.
Put another sheet on top and leave to cool for about 15 minutes. Using a sharp knife cut into squares.

A good alternative to after dinner chocolates for a dinner
party and a gift, wrapped in a paper doily or gift paper, tied
with a ribbon.

Childrens' parties (gluten-free)

These seems to have become more organized over the years
instead of an overexcited free-for-all. Instead of a table full of
food on plates each child can be given a little box with a
selection of food. Large celebration cakes seem to have have
been superseded by the cup cake – sugary, over-decorated and
very popular. Leftover food goes out of the door in 'goody

bags'. There's no washing up as the boxes go into the bin. Fruit juice or what they would like is the rule as regards drinks.

To make cup cakes, make the sponge buns in chapter 10. Top with water icing and decorate with icing squiggles in a different colour, or names– again, use water icing. (Cake decorations seem to have been the target for non gluten-free decorations – a kind of sugar made from wheat seemingly has taken over from cane and beet sugar. Avoid these unless you are sure they are gluten-free.)

Adults' Buffet (gluten-free)
Start with nibbles (see above) and a drink.

A cold collation – plates of plain roasted cold meat – beef, chicken, ham (without breadcrumb coating) – cold salmon – salads – potato salad – a showy dessert – strawberry tartlets – gluten-free French bread (see chapter 3) – fruit salad – sherry, wines, coffee and tea. Lay all the food out attractively on large plates so people can help themselves easily with serviettes and cutlery. See chapters 8 and 10 for starters, salads and desserts as well as this chapter. This is a chance to show that gluten-free food can be wonderful.

Dinner parties
For the gluten-free dieter this kind of dining is much safer than dining out. A formal, sit-down meal with a soup or starter, main meal and dessert is what will please most people. Make it colourful. Make at least two of the courses ones which can be made ahead. Present it well and take trouble with how you dress the table. Put a small vase of flowers on the table, cloth napkins, place mats or a table cloth. Candles always create a relaxing mood and are kinder than too much electric light. Don't give up on all this just because the meal is gluten-free. Be proud and do it justice.

Obviously it is easier for the cook if everything throughout the meal is gluten-free without different food for the gluten-free dieters. All the following are from this book. You will need gluten-free chocolates from a store, or make the nougat from this chapter.

*Menu A * denotes special gluten-free*

    parma ham and melon
    *pasta with a *meat sauce and a green side salad
    *profiteroles or exotic fruit salad
    *chocolates and coffee or tea

Menu B

    *soup
    grilled or baked fish or grilled meat with a *sauce and
        hot vegetables (one green), including boiled new
        potatoes
    *Pear and chocolate upside down pudding or fruit salad
    *crispbreads and cheeses with celery or apples and
        *chutney

Tea party

    *scones, jam and whipped cream
    *Lemon and yoghurt cake
    exotic fruit salad or a bowl of strawberries or raspberries
    *moon biscuits

Entertaining pushes the boat out so that the healthy gluten-free food normally on the table becomes forgotten for an hour or two. This is gluten-free feasting and it is not meant to be the selection of food to eat everyday. However, once in awhile it probably won't do any harm *as long as it is gluten free.* Never go over the top and break the gluten-free regime as it is quite likely to lash back and make you ill. Coming off the diet is silly – you can have gorgeous gluten-free food with a bit of effort.

Celebration – buffet lunch or supper

As it doesn't hurt anyone, why not put a complete gluten-free buffet on the table? Easiest is a cold buffet where people can help themselves. This will involve some easy dishes to eat with cold meats or fish and a couple of showy desserts. It can make a colourful table. Here is a suggested spread and it is all gluten-free.

Welcome

    Vegetable dips and nibbles to have with drinks – see chapter 5

    Wine and alcoholic drinks, spring water and fruit juices

Main course

    cold chicken (roasted)

    cold ham (without breadcrumb coating)

    cold poached salmon

    hard boiled eggs, shelled

    bowl of grated cheese

    bowl of prawns in gluten-free light mayonnaise

    large dish of potato salad with gluten-free mayonnaise and chives (see chapter 8)

    rice salad with vinaigrette (see chapter 8)

    purple salad with vinaigrette

    green salad without dressing

    plate of cucumber slices

    bowl of light mayonnaise

Desserts
    bowl of exotic fruit salad – see chapter 9
    gateaux – see this chapter
    Pavlova

Finish
    Gluten-free chocolates (bought)
    Gluten-free nougat – see recipe in this chapter
    coffee and tea to finish with the confectionary

(There is no need to tell everyone that is a gluten-free event. When they have enjoyed all the food and had a good time, then is the time to tell them. They will be amazed as most people believe that gluten-free food has to be dire and generate sympathy. Show them this is nonsense.)

Iced buns/water icing No stars at all!
Any of the plain sponge buns in chapter 10 can be iced with water icing. Put 4 level tablespoons icing sugar into basin and add 1 teaspoon of water plus a few drops. Mix to a cream and use a knife to spread over the tops of the buns. For chocolate flavour add 1 teaspoon cocoa. For orange and lemon add 1 level teaspoon finely grated orange or lemon peel. For pink icing add a few drops of beetroot juice.

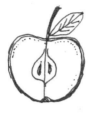

CHAPTER 13

Nutrition and Healthy Gluten-free Eating

Taking the gluten out of your diet can be quite difficult at first as gluten turns up in many foods. To remove it all at once can be quite traumatic and requires a burst of energy and resolve to reorganize your food/eating, to change your cooking skills and rethink your shopping.

There may be a large gap caused at first by not eating wheat – bread, rolls, breakfast cereals, cakes, pastries, pasta, pizza, scones, biscuits etc, etc. It is a big ask. The realization that the situation is life changing can be quite a shock and although the promise is much better health, it doesn't work out that way if you don't understand what needs to be sorted out and why. Sudden change is never easy but it is not impossible.

What does a healthy body require in the way of food? The answer is protein, fats, fibre, carbohydrate, water, vitamins, minerals and micronutrients (trace elements). These foods don't arrive in every food just on their own but generally in a mixture. The body has to digest the foods and then use them for energy, movement, work, growth, repair (and sometimes reproduction). The digestive system breaks down the food chemically and passes it into the bloodstream which can take it all round the body to where it is needed. Solid waste is passed out and so is waste liquid.

In the Western world we enjoy what is called a 'mixed diet'. We have access to a wide variety of foods from all over the world, not just what can be produced in the area where we live. This enables us to take in everything we need for our bodies to function well and for us to be healthy. However, our digestion needs to be in good order to cope with our food intake, otherwise it will pass through us and be wasted.

When gluten cannot be digested properly the result can be poor health. Babies and children may fail to thrive and grow. Adults can just become ill and weak. The fact that gluten can have such a bad effect on the health of *some* is extraordinary but it does happen. The good news is that by cutting gluten completely out of the diet, health can be restored as the digestion begins to function properly again and children can thrive and grow as they should, without pills or drugs.

Essentials for a healthy diet

Protein is needed for energy, growth and repair. Good sources are plain lean meat, fish, eggs, dried milk, and cheese. (By coincidence all these are gluten-free).

Carbohydrate is mainly needed for energy. In an ordinary diet this would mean wheat but there is also sugar which is very high in carbohydrates and not a good idea in large amounts, whatever the diet.

Fat is a high energy food. It also helps with body function. In can be stored in the body and made from excess protein, carbohydrate and fat from food. It enables us to have a constant source of energy, however, something simple like eating too much food can cause the store of body fat becoming much too large, leading to obesity. The body can become too much for its skeleton frame and muscles. Health problems can result. Life becomes uncomfortable.

Fat comes into the diet from butter, cream, milk, cheeses, margarine, nuts and oils – such as sunflower, olive, corn etc and the fat in/on meat, lard etc. There are different kinds of fat – saturated including cholesterol (as in butter), polyunsaturated (as in sunflower oil) and monounsaturated (as in olive oil).

Fibre is used by the digestive system to make passing out of waste food easy.

In an ordinary diet wheat bran (which is not gluten-free) would be important but there are also beans, peas, root and leafy vegtables, sweetcorn (maize), dried fruit and fresh fruit with pips, skins and seeds e.g. raspberries and tomatoes (all gluten-free).

Water is essential for life. Body tissue cannot store very much water and we need to keep topping it up especially as two thirds of our body weight is water.

Vitamins, minerals and micronutrients (trace elements) are necessary for efficient working of the body. They are found in many foods and fruit and vegetables are a good source. (By coincidence, all fruit and vegetables are gluten-free.) Important nutrients in wheat-gluten are iron, zinc, B1, B2, B3 and Vitamin E. If wheat is removed from the diet these should be put back in. Some people might need a vitamin and mineral supplement to help them adjust when starting a gluten-free diet. Pharmacies should be able to recommend a brand that is gluten-free. Most tablets have a filler and it isn't always gluten-free. The pharmacist can look it up and advise you. When you have sorted out the gluten-free diet and balanced it there will probably be no need for the supplement.

Obesity. Too much of some foods, particularly fat and carbohydrate can result in obesity. The excess food converts to fat for storage in the body to be used at a later date. However, with the continuation of overeating the later date does not arrive and the body keeps adding to the fat stores. The body becomes heavier and heavier.

Starvation is the result of the lack of food which in turn leads to deficiencies in vitamins and minerals, a loss of stored body fat and even wasting of muscles. Movement becomes difficult due to lack of energy, no repair can take place and no new cells can be made. If the lack of food goes on too long the result is death, as sometimes happens in anorexia.

Calories. With a ruler you can measure the size of something. With calories you can work out what the energy value of a food is. e.g a packet of crisps has an energy value of about 115 calories. Calories are not a kind of food but a kind of measurement. The average man needs 2,500 calories worth of food every day, a woman 2000, small growing children need less and older growing children need more. To lose 1lb (500g) of fat you will need to burn up about 3,500 calories.

Changes in balance for a gluten-free diet

The average Western everyday diet is far from perfect. Most people eat too much fat, salt and sugar but not enough fruit vegetables or fibre. The same mistakes can be made on a gluten-free diet. It has been going on for many years.

Without wheat and the foods made from it, other high carbohydrate foods need to be substituted. Potatoes, rice and bananas are all useful. Gluten-free breakfast cereals based on maize (sweetcorn), rice and millet (see health food stores and 'free-from' sections in supermarkets) and gluten-free food you can easily make yourself at home will help to bridge the gap. You will find recipes to help throughout this book. Don't fall into the trap of thinking that every manufactured food labeled 'gluten-free' will make you well. It may be just gluten-free junk food.

Basic Daily Guide – foods for a healthy gluten-free diet

Carbohydrate – 3 – 4 portions, choose from gluten-free: bread, pasta, crispbreads, pancakes, rice porridge, breakfast cereals, pizza, biscuits, potatoes, rice – see recipes for lots more.

Greens – very important every day 1 – 2 portions – choose from green cabbage, spinach, kale, watercress, spring greens, green lettuce, broccoli, Brussels sprouts.

Other fresh and frozen, plain vegetables – 4 portions – onions, carrots, leeks, green beans, swede, parsnips, turnips, celeriac, beetroot, courgettes, peppers, tomatoes, salad vegetables, radishes, celery, corn-on-the-cob, cucumber, fennel, asparagus etc.

Fresh and frozen fruit – 3 portions – apples, oranges, pears, bananas, pineapple, grapes, strawberries, raspberries, blackcurrants, redcurrants, peaches, nectarines, apricots, plums, melon, kiwi, avocado, papaya, cherries, summer fruit mixtures etc.

High protein – 2-3 portions – plain meat, fish, gluten-free TVP, prawns, crab and shellfish, gluten-free tofu, plain nuts, low-fat cheeses.

Fats and oils (except wheatgerm oil) – 2 tablespoons – sunflower oil, extra virgin olive oil, polyunsaturated soft margarines, butter (a little).

Sugar – 1 tablespoon or less – choose from sugar, jam, honey, golden syrup

Salt – up to 6 grams for an adult, less for a child

Milk – ¼ pint (150ml) – low fat milk (adults) – if cows' milk cannot be tolerated use other milks, children will need more than this.

Treats – 1 small portion – a gluten-free biscuit or piece of cake, gluten-free chocolate or sweet, snacks – see recipes.

See chapter14 for information on oats.

Balance
To help you understand the difference between a poor gluten-free diet and a healthy one, here are two charts. You can see how different they are.

DIET BALANCE

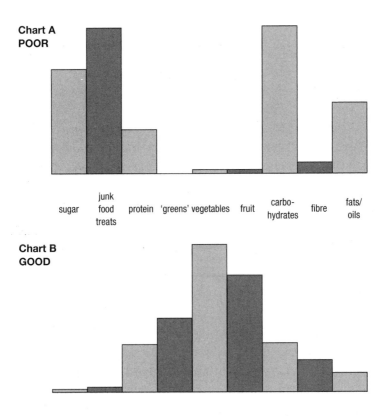

Chart A – a poor gluten-free diet with far too little fruit and vegetables, too much fat and sugar, a great deal of junk food and no greens.

Chart B – a good gluten-free diet with plenty of fruit and vegetables, greens and the right amount of carbohydrate with minimal junkfood.

In a well-balanced gluten-free diet the part that is affected by having to be turned into gluten-free is a mere **one fifth of the diet**. In a badly balanced gluten-free diet it would be **most of it.**

The reason we all need a diet with a lot of variety is so that we can have access to vitamins, minerals and trace elements. The worst supply of these is in junk foods. This list will give you some idea of what is required in a healthy diet.

A few vitamins and minerals can be stored in the body but most need to be taken in in a regular supply. Exposure to the sun causes vitamin D to be made in the body. Vitamins A,D, E and F are built into fats and they are found in animal and fish oils. An excellent source of vitamins and minerals is fresh vegetables and fruit.

Vitamins – what are they for?

Vitamin A for healthy bones, hair, eyes, skin, teeth.

Vitamin B complex (B1,B2, B6, B12) for healthy eyes, food canal, hair, brain, ears, heart, nervous system, nails, liver, skin, blood, muscles, gall bladder, glands, tongue.

Biotin for cell growth, for making fat, for helping to use protein, fat and carbohydrate in the body.

Choline for a healthy liver, gall bladder and nerves.

Folic acid for the appetite, reproduction, circulation, liver function, red blood cell formation.

Inositol for helping to stop the arteries from hardening, for reducing cholesterol, for helping the body to use fat and grow hair.

Niacin for healthy circulation, for sex hormone production, for helping the body to use protein, fat and carbohydrate.

PABA (para-aminobenzoic acid) for healthy hair and skin.

Pantothenic acid for helping to remove toxic substances, for possibly helping hair to keep its colour, for activating friendly bacteria in the food canal and helping the body to use protein.

Vitamin C for healthy adrenal glands, blood, skin, ligaments, bones, gums, heart and teeth.

Vitamin D for healthy bones, heart, nerves, skin, teeth, thyroid gland.

Vitamin F (polyunsaturated fatty acids) for healthy cells, glands, hair, nerves, skin.

Vitamin E for healthy blood vessels, heart, lungs, nerves, skin.

Vitamin K for healthy blood and liver.

Vitamin P (bioflavonoids) for healthy blood, skin, gums, ligaments, bones, teeth.

Minerals – what are they for?

Calcium for healthy bones, blood, heart, skin, teeth.

Chromium for blood circulation.

Copper for healthy blood, bones, circulation, hair and skin.

Iodine for hair, nails, skin, teeth, thyroid gland.

Iron for healthy blood, bones, nails and skin.

Magnesium for healthy arteries, bones, heart, muscles, nerves, teeth.

Manganese for healthy brain, muscles, nerves.

Phosphorus for healthy bones, blood, brain, nerves, teeth.

Potassium for healthy blood, heart, kidneys, muscles, nerves, skin.

Selenium for a healthy pancreas.

Sodium for healthy blood, muscles and nerves.

Zinc for healthy blood, heart.

Good sources of vitamins for a gluten-free diet

Vitamin A – fish, fish liver oil, green and yellow fruit and vegetables, carrots, spinach.

Vitamin B1 – brewer's yeast, yoghurt

Vitamin B2 – brewer's yeast, eggs, fruit, green vegetables leaves, beans, nuts, poultry.

Vitamin B6 – avocado pears, bananas, brewer's yeast, cabbage, fish green vegetable leaves, prunes, raisins, walnuts.

Vitamin B12 – beef, eggs, milk products, fish, pork, cottage cheese.

Biotin – brewer's yeast, egg yolk, beans.

Choline – brewer's yeast, egg yolk, fish, beans, soya.

Folic acid – oranges, lemons, eggs, green vegetable leaves, milk products, seafood.

Inositol – brewer's yeast, oranges, lemons, meat, milk, nuts, vegetables.

Niacin – eggs, lean meat, milk products, poultry, seafood.

PABA – brewer's yeast, eggs, liver, milk, rice, yeast, brown rice, eggs, sunflower and sesame seeds.

Pantothenic acid – brewer's yeast, eggs, beans, mushrooms, salmon.

Vitamin C – fresh fruit and vegetables.

Vitamin D – egg yolk, milk, fish, fishbones (as in canned salmon).

Vitamin E – butter, dark green vegetable leaves e.g. kale and spinach, eggs, fruit, nuts, vegetable oils.

Vitamin F – safflower, sunflower corn and soya oils, sunflower seeds.

Vitamin K – green vegetable leaves, safflower oil, yoghurt.

Vitamin P – fruits including skin – apricots, grapes, cherries, grapefruit, plums, lemons.

Good sources of minerals for a gluten-free diet

Calcium – milk, cheese, yoghurt, almonds

Chromium – brewer's yeast, corn oil.

Copper – beans, nuts, seafood, raisins, avocado, liver, soya, beansprouts, watercress, parsley.

Iodine – seafood, seaweed.

Iron – eggs, fish, poultry, liver, dark green vegetables, spices.

Magnesium – honey, green vegetables, nuts.

Manganese – bananas, celery, egg yolks, green vegetable leaves, beans, liver, nuts, pineapple.

Phosphorus – dates, figs, meat, poultry, liver.

Potassium – dates, figs, peaches, tomatoes, raisins, seafood, sunflower seeds, fresh vegetables, fresh fruit.

Selenium – fish, meat, eggs, brown rice.

Sodium – salt, milk, cheese, seafood.

Zinc – brewer's yeast, liver, seafood, soya, mushrooms, sunflower seeds, spinach.

You can see from these lists that junkfoods are conspicuous by their absence. Salt and potassium form a balance in our bodies. Most of us eat far too much salt and too little potassium. Salt can be reduced by not taking too much at table and avoiding excessively salty foods. Potassium can be increased by eating more fresh fruit and vegetables.

Trends in eating
After the second world war, rationing in the UK went on for years. It took until the mid fifties before the shortages stopped and supermarkets began. Suddenly there was a lot more food available and moderation went out of the window. Cookery books began to emerge, in full colour, full of exciting foreign food. Junk food began to take a hold as sugar and fat became cheap and the snack market took off. Gradually the demand for convenience food grew. as people became disconnected from home cooking. Schools took domestic science and cookery off the curriculum. The media began to take an interest and chefs and cooks began to have their own cult programmes on TV. The actual food began to take a back seat as displays of temperament, strange recipes with many ingredients, expensive gadgetry and exotic ideas expanded the world of food. By the second decade of the 21st century, the average diet had become too high in salt, fat and sugar, too low in fibre and a sure way to obesity for nearly half the population, with all its health risks and problems. Lifestyle and self became very important, in fact more important than health and food. Rumblings began about the dire situation but

that is all – just rumblings. The cult of celebrity took over from knowledge and skill as the key to eating well. Cookery books, once a mine of commonsense and simple, nourishing food, became full of amazing colour photographs. In fact they tended to be more about colour photography and the fame of the author than actual food. Spin offs are restaurants, TV series and merchandise to sell. The plot has been well and truly lost. Food seems to be for entertainment and feasting rather than something essential for good health.

There is no shortage of food in the western world. Half of all food produced is just wasted. Farmers are under ever more pressure to produce more from the land as the population expands. Perhaps if there was a shortage, people would be more careful about what they eat and more inclined to eat for their health instead of just feasting and entertainment.

Easiest to follow gluten-free diet
This might help people just beginning or it can be the way some people cope.

Breakfast – gluten-free breakfast cereal such as cornflakes from 'free from' shelves of a supermarket or health store, fresh fruit, **or,** egg and tomato with fried cold boiled potato.

Lunch – hot or cold potato, salad with gluten-free dressing, cold plain cooked meat, fish, or low fat cheese, fresh fruit.

Main meal – plain roast or grilled chicken, beef, pork, lamb, **or,** omelet or plain fish/prawns with plain boiled potatoes/ rice and steamed vegetables, one of which should be green and leafy. Stewed or fresh fruit.

Snacks – dried fruit and nuts, banana.

Extras – butter, margarine, single cream, plain unflvoured yoghurt, plain cheese.

No bread, rolls, cakes, biscuits, sweets, chocolate, junkfood snacks, gravy.

Gluten-free lifestyle
While some people settle down to their new gluten-free lifestyle, others do not and forever hold a grudge about it. This makes it difficult for family and friends..

Other people go on diets of gluten-free food from the supermarket expensive 'free-from' shelves and spend hours studying labels on packets – anything rather than cook at home. If you know what to do, gluten-free is an easy diet to follow, but it should be done in a healthy way. The most wonderful advantage anyone can have in life is good health. Go for it.

Stars
To help you sort out the **health value** of the recipes in this handbook, you will find stars awarded. Here is what they mean.

***** very good
**** good
*** quite good
** poor
* not very good at all

The recipes in chapter12 are the ones for feasting, not everyday food. Notice the lack of stars. This is a chapter to cook from now and then, not every day. Life would be a misery if we didn't eat the occasional treat, however, this is not the kind of food to live on. On any special diet it is important to eat in a healthy way. This doesn't mean your food should be boring. On the contrary, to make you keep to the special diet it should be interesting, attractive, nutritious and and colourful even if it is gluten-free.

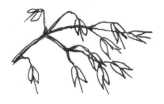

CHAPTER 14

Oats and Miscellaneous

Because oats have a slightly different form of gluten than wheat, rye and barley, some coeliacs are now allowed them. This has come about after trials on coeliacs in Scandinavia at the end of the 20th century. Not everyone is able to take oats.

The idea is not as exciting as it sounds as oats contain avenin, a weak kind of protein. This is nothing like as good as wheat gluten so oats are rather limited regarding perform-ance in baking. Meusli, oatcakes, flapjacks, treacle tart, melting moments and porridge really wrap it up and are clas-sic oat recipes. Oats can be used in with wheat for mixed grain bread but have not taken the world by storm yet. On the positive side, oat flour is very easy to make in a coffee grinder or mini food processor and can be mixed into recipes instead of all wheat flour. This means it should mix into a homemade gluten-free blend. However, not much can be achieved with it as it is soft (because it has been processed) and a weak binder – nothing like as good as wheat.

Another problem with oats for a gluten-free diet is con-tamination with wheat as it is processed in factories/mills that also handle wheat. A source of oats from a dedicated mill needs to be used. They can be bought from health stores or 'free-from' sections. The price is higher than ordinary oats and they are not always easy to come by. This tends to put people off. In the body, oats give a slow release of energy which really means they might not be easily digested by some people with digestive problems.

Oats are undoubtedly good for us if we can digest them. They are nutritious and have a very characteristic taste and texture.

*Oats should not be included in a gluten-free diet without first consulting a medical practitioner. The oats used should be from **a dedicated source,** not just bought off the super-market shelf, as these will probably be contaminated by wheat.*

For those who can take oats, here are a few simple recipes where oats are combined with a gluten-free flour blend and the usual gluten-free binders.

Oats on their own will not make a loaf of bread, alas. Nor will they make pastry or shaped baking. However, for those who are allowed them they can make a welcome addition to strict gluten-free diet. (Some people on an ordinary diet never take to them and they don't suit everybody so be prepared for this.)

Oat flour is best made just before you want to use it. Weigh out the oats then blitz in a mini-food processor or coffee grinder. Food baked with oats tends to be crumbly as its version of gluten (avenin) is very weak.

There is no special kind of oats for people on a gluten-free diet (except those processed in a dedicated mill). Oats can take many forms – groats, the actual oat grain, is processed to make porridge oats or oatmeal. Oat bran and oat germ are used for sprinkling over breakfast cereals. Grinding groats results in oatmeal. There are three grades –

pinhead (coarse), medium and fine. They are more difficult to digest and take much longer to cook than porridge oats, which are also known as oatflakes, flaked oats, rolled oats, superfast oats, quick oats and easy oats. They are heat treated and rolled to flatten them, which is why they don't take so long to cook. There are also jumbo oats, which are rolled large and thin, and small oats which are just small porridge oats.

'Instant oats' are the most processed form of oats. By adding hot water or milk, the smooth porridge it produces is instant. The convenience of it makes it popular and it can have added vitamins and minerals. Although it looks like weaning food for babies it is not suitable for this task. It should not be used for babies as they are not able to digest it. Oats can be processed to make oat milk which is popular with vegans. This can also be bought as flavoured oat milks.

If you are using oats, don't store them for too long. They don't keep anything like as well as wheat flour. Buy little and often and store in a cool, dry place. If you have not used them after three months, throw them away and buy fresh.

Whatever kind of oat products you buy, if you are allowed them on your gluten-free diet, always check the label. Do they come from a dedicated mill and packing factory? Is there a warning on the packet that they are not suitable?

Muesli
See chapter 4 for this recipe. Use raw rolled oats instead of the cooked rice.

Oat coating *****
Make oat flour and use instead of breadcrumbs for coating fishcakes – see chapter 7. However, they may not be to your taste as they can be rather 'mealy'.

Oatcakes (makes 8) *****
This is an example of a kind of crispbread which has some oats and some gluten-free flour in them, as opposed to all oats.
Good, crunchy biscuits to eat with cheese or soup. Commercial versions of these are heavy on salt to give them a longer shelf life.

2 oz (50g) rolled oats made into flour
½ oz (15g) RG77 gluten-free flour blend
1 pinch bicarbonate of soda
2 pinches salt
1 tablespoon sunflower oil
1 tablespoon boiling water from the kettle
rice flour for kneading

Preheat oven at Gas 5/190°C/375°F. Cut a piece of baking parchment to line a baking tray. Blitz the oats to make into flour. Put into a bowl with the flour, bicarbonate of soda and salt. Mix well and add the oil. Stir with a fork then add the hot water. Bring the mixture together by hand into 1 sticky lump of dough. Knead for 30 seconds after sprinkling with rice flour. Use more to dust the baking parchment. Put the baking parchment on to the worktop and put the dough into the middle of it. Sprinkle with rice flour and roll out into a circle. Transfer to the baking tray, still on the baking parchment. Use a sharp knife to cut in half then quarters. Cut each quarter in half to make a total of 8 wedges.

Bake on the top shelf for about 35 minutes, until browning. Leave on the tray for 3 minutes then move to a wire rack to grow cold and crisp. Store in an airtight container. Good with cheese.

Oat porridge (1 serving) *****
Put 3 level tablespoons rolled oats into a small saucepan with a just over a cup of water or milk and water. Get out any lumps. Bring gently to the boil and simmer for 4 minutes, while you stir. Turn into a serving bowl. Serve hot with a little skimmed milk and sprinkled with demerara sugar.

Oat and honey breakfast flakes (makes 1 serving or 2 with fruit) ***

> 3 level tablespoons rolled oats
> 1 generous teaspoon runny honey
> 1 level teaspoon caster sugar
> 1 pinch salt
> 4 tablespoons water

Method: Preheat oven at Gas 8/230°C/450° F. Grind the oats to a fine powder in a coffee grinder. Put into a basin with the remaining ingredients and mix/beat to a smooth, thin batter. Have ready a large baking sheet lined with baking parchment. Leaving space between, put little blobs of the batter on the sheet – a teaspoon will make 3 flakes. Bake on the top shelf for about 7 minutes, until brown round the edges. Cool for a minute then peel off and leave to cool in a cereal plate for 5 minutes. Eat on their own with skimmed milk or with fruit such as sliced strawberries, banana, or raspberries. If you can't face making these first thing in the morning, make them the night before. DIY breakfast cereal – what could be nicer?

Flapjacks (makes 12 bars) No stars at all
As this is a classic oat recipe it can be seen as a very early form of sticky, chewy junkfood. They contain a large amount of sugar and syrup which sticks the oats together. It illustrates

how a healthy food like oats can become something quite the
opposite with additions.

2 oz (50g) polyunsaturated soft margarine
2 oz (50g) golden syrup (warm the spoon)
4 oz (100g) demerara sugar
6 oz (170g) rolled oats

Method: Preheat oven at Gas 4/160°C/350°F. Put the margarine, syrup and sugar into a saucepan and set over a gentle
heat. Stir while the margarine melts and the sugar dissolves.
Take off the heat and stir in the oats. Have ready an 8 in
(20cm) square tin, lined with baking parchment. Turn the
mixture into it and spread flat with the back of a metal spoon.
Bake on the top shelf for about 20 minutes until golden
brown. Leave in the tin for 5 minutes, then cut into 12 bars
with a sharp knife, making sure you cut right through. Leave
in the tin to grow cold. Turn up side down and peel off the
baking parchment. Store in an airtight tin, wrapped individually in food film.

Note: Use 1 oz (25g) less oats and add 1oz(25g) chopped
nuts – cashews, hazelnuts, walnuts, almonds are all suitable.

Sweet mincemeat for mincepies ****
Early versions of this traditional Christmas pie filling actually
contained meat. Commercial versions still do in the form of
suet which is usually rolled in wheat flour to keep the pieces
of suet from clumping together. Try this gluten-free version –
it couldn't be simpler.

3 oz (75g) each of sultanas and currants
2 oz (50g) each of raisins and chopped almonds
2 oz (50g) soft brown sugar
1 medium apple, finely grated

½ teaspoon each of allspice, ground cinnamon and grated
  nutmeg
finely grated rind of 1 lemon
2 oz (50g) melted margarine
1 tablespoon brandy
fresh orange juice

Method: Put all the ingredients except the orange juice into a
bowl and mix well. Add enough orange juice to moisten –
about 1 tablespoon. Put into clean jars, label and date. Store
in the fridge until required. Keeps well. Use all the year
round.

Quick apple chutney ***
Makes 1 small jar. It only takes a few minutes to make, unlike
most chutney which can take 2 hours or more.

1 cooking apple, peeled and cored
1 small onion, peeled and chopped small
1 heaped tablespoon soft brown sugar
4 pinches ground ginger
3 stoned dates or 1 heaped tablespoon sultanas
3 tablespoons wine vinegar

Method: Grate the apple and put into a small pan with the
other ingredients. Cook while you stir for about 10 minutes,
until the apple is soft. Put into a clean jar, cover and store in
the fridge. Label and date it.

Brandy butter No stars at all.
Commercial versions of this are not so simple and may not
be gluten-free. This one is and can be served to the whole
family.

4 oz (100g) unsalted butter
6 oz (175g) icing sugar
4 tablespoons brandy

Method: Put the butter into a warmed bowl, cut into small cubes. Cream with a wooden spoon until soft and light. Put the icing sugar on a plate and press out any lumps with a spoon. Gradually beat the sugar into the creamed butter with the brandy. Cover and store in the fridge. Use with Christmas pudding and mincepies.

Stuffing ***

Savoury stuffings to eat with pork and poultry are usually on a base of wheat breadcrumbs with onion and herbs. You can use gluten-free bread to make the crumbs or use cooked rice. Serve to everyone or make a special small dish for the gluten-free dieter. Herbs and onion are gluten-free so it is only the base that is the problem. Popular stuffings are sage and onion and mixed herb. Make them all in the same way. Mix the base of gluten-free breadcrumbs (made in a coffee grinder) or cooked rice with a finely chopped small onion and a tablespoon of sunflower oil. Add the herb(s) of your choice, salt and freshly ground black pepper to taste. Mix well and turn into a small, greased oven-proof dish. Bake in the oven the same time as the roast meat, on the top shelf. It should be ready after 30 minutes – crisp and brown. Move down to the bottom of the oven to keep warm until you are ready to serve. Here are three versions.

Sage and onion – add 4 fresh sage leaves, finely chopped or ½ a teaspoon dried.
For pork or chicken.
Lemon and thyme – add a few sprigs of fresh thyme, 4 pinches of dried and the finely grated rind of ½ a lemon. For chicken.

Mixed herbs – add 1 teaspoon fresh mixed herbs – rosemary, thyme, sage, or ½ a teaspoon dried. If using with pork, add ½ a finely grated eating apple.

Milkshakes ***

These are best made with low fat milk, so dried milk can be used. Sugar or honey is added to taste but should not overpower the fruit. To increase the protein a little ground almond can be added. It all depends on the purpose of the drink. Is it to make someone put on weight? Does it replace food for someone who doesn't want to (or can't) eat solid food?

Flavours

Banana – 1 cup water,1 teaspoon runny honey, 1 heaped tablespoon dried milk granules, ½ a banana.

Berries – 1 cup water, 1 heaped tablespoon dried milk granules, handful of strawberries or raspberries, a little caster sugar to taste. Put into a liquidizer and blend. Pour into a tumbler and serve immediately.

Other fruits to use are:

- 6 dried apricots, soaked in water overnight
- ½ a ripe peach or nectarine, de-stoned
- 2 ripe dessert plums, de-stoned
- 8 de-stoned cherries
- 1 peeled kiwi fruit
- 1 fresh pineapple ring, chopped
- ½ an eating apple, peeled and cored
- 3 prunes, stones removed

Lemonade **

Lemon barley water is not allowed on a gluten-free diet because of the barley, but this substitute is and can be diluted and used instead of squash. Because it is made with fresh fruit, the flavour of the lemons is very intense. Good for when people have a cold or flu and in hot weather.

2 lemons
2 tablespoons caster sugar
about 1½ pints(900 ml) boiling water from the kettle

Method: Wash the fruit and put on to a board to cut into thin slices. Put into a jug and pour over the water. Leave to steep, covered, for about 12 hours. Drain through a sieve into a bowl. (Discard the lemon slices.) Stir in the sugar. Pour into a bottle or jar and keep in the fridge to use as required. Label and date it.

Specially for children – exciting breads
For children, the **Coburg** loaves, baps and round rolls from chapter 3 can be slashed before they rise.

Smiley face loaf and rolls – cut with a sharp knife as shown.

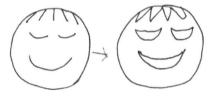

Crocodile bread and crocodile baps can be made by snipping with kitchen scissors as shown. Do this before leaving the loaf to rise.

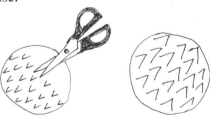

Hedgehog bread – shape the bread as shown, making a cut for the mouth. A raisin pressed in will make an eye. The spines can be made by snipping the dough with kitchen scissors, in curved lines. Do this before leaving the bread to rise.

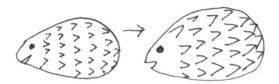

Breadsticks can be made in short lengths, more suitable for children. Roll them just as long as a finger before leaving to rise. Make them all the same length if you can.

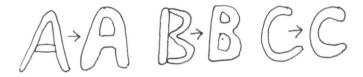

Alphabet bread
As the dough is easy to shape, initial letters are a possibility. Roll into long sausages first and then shape. Bake for less time.

Child's gluten-free happy face dinner
A distraction, a novelty, a nonsense – anything to get a child to eat a meal. Something special can be put together out of ordinary gluten-free food. (It is important to get children to eat vegetables. If they won't they may go all their lives without them and suffer the consequences.)

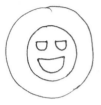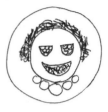

Make a happy face on a plate. Spread cooked rice or mashed potato in a circle and remove, *right through to the plate,* two half circular holes for the eyes and a shape for the mouth. Fill the eyes with peas and the mouth with chopped tomato. For the hair use chopped green beans, spinach or sweetcorn. Make a necklace with cut up cooked meat/fish or round carrot slices.

Note: Avoid circles for the eyes as this will make it look like a skull! However, some children would love this.

****

Eggs

The recipes in this book that contain eggs are not suitable for use with egg replacer.

Very fresh, new-laid eggs are not suitable for baking. Eggs that are at least a week old will be fine.

Candied Peel

Trying to buy candied peel which is gluten/wheat-free is difficult. There are three ways round the problem.

1. Omit the candied peel and use tiny cubes of dried apricots. Cut each apricot into strips then cut across to make the cubes as shown. To make up for the flavour of candied peel use grated rinds of orange and lemon.

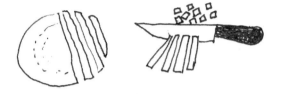

2. This solution takes time but can work well. Peel an orange and a lemon with a serrated knife so that you take off the pith with the peel. Cut into long thin strips. Put into a pan with 2 cups of water and bring to the boil. Lower heat to a simmer and continue to cook for about an hour or more until the rinds are soft. Give them a stir from time to time and don't let the water get too low. (Top it up with a little boiling water from the kettle if it does.] When the rinds are soft, take them out with a slotted spoon and put on to a board. Allow to cool enough to handle, then holding 3 or 4 strips together, cut across to make tiny cubes. Put back into the pan with about a tablespoon of what is left of the water and add a tablespoon of caster sugar. Stir over a low heat to dissolve the sugar. Spoon into a clean jar and put on the lid. Keep in the fridge until required.
Note: They will still be chewy so make sure you make small cubes.

3. Empty a jar or chunky style marmalade on to a plate. Pick out the pieces of citrus peel and chop. Use instead of candied peel. This is an expensive way of making it but you can still use the jelly part of the marmalade.

Skin conditions

Something wrong inside can reveal itself by something amiss on the outside - the skin. Rightly or wrongly, gluten intolerance has been linked to several skin conditions such as eczema, psoriasis, dermatitis herpetiformis, dry skin and acne. Going on to a gluten-free diet that is not properly balanced will not help but a balanced, healthy one might lead to improvement.

The Invisible Enemy – Gluten

This list gives an idea of where the invisible enemy gluten lurks. Notice how much there is in the bakery section. This is because the basis for these foods is wheat, the major source of gluten in our diet. Most of the items will be bought and a few will be made at home.

Bakery products: (food made with flour)
wheat/rye/barley bread, loaves, rolls, cakes, scones, buns, sponges, cookies, pastry, pastries, bars, brownies, doughnuts, bagels, biscuits, slices, crispbreads, water biscuits, biscuits for cheese, choux buns and eclairs, croissants, muffins, drop-scones, pancakes, pikelets, crumpets, teacakes, burger buns, baps, cupcakes, fruit cakes, par-baked bread, dumplings, cia-batta, baguettes, pitta, wraps, tacos, pasties, pies, tarts, sausage rolls, macaroons, straws, dumplings, spelt bread, soda bread

Breakfast cereals:
puffs, flakes, bars, granolas, mueslis etc.

Confectionery:
sweets, chocolates, bars, toffees etc.

Pasta: (food made with semolina and flour)
spaghetti, tagliatelle, noodles, lasagna sheets, shaped pastas, ravioli, gnocci,

Stock:
stock cubes, liquid stocks, powdered stocks, stock and gravy mixes, cooking sauces, curry powder and sauces.

Soups:
canned, frozen, in cartons

Snacks:
flavoured crisps, nibbles, dips, straws, coated nuts etc.

Sauces etc.:
gravies, sweet sauces, savoury sauces, tables sauces, custard, toppings, dressings, mayonnaises, cream substitutes, marinades, relishes, chutneys, spreads, fillings, dips, cook-in sauces

Desserts:
puddings, pies, tarts, trifles, ice creams, yoghurts, custards, caramels

Meat:
corned beef, processed meat, sausages, meat loaves, casseroles and stews, pies, meat in breadcrumb coatings

Fish:
in batter and breadcrumbs, canned in sauce

Drinks:
bedtime drinks, hot chocolate etc.

Finishings/decorations:
icings, marzipans, coatings, sprays, cake decorations

Mixes:
pancakes, batters, coatings, crumbles, pastry, bread etc.

Flours:
Bread flour, strong flour, multigrain, brown, white, wholemeal, wholewheat, spelt, rye, barley, self-raising flour

Miscellaneous:
Ready meals – mains and sides, baby food, teething rusks, prepared raw vegetable mixes, salad bags with sprouting seeds. If you want to buy any of these you must check the labels carefully to make sure what you are buying is gluten-free. Remember, all naturally gluten-free foods will be unprocessed.

Recipe Index

Nutrition/Health and General Index